# SECRETS OF
# INDIAN MEDICINE

Dr. R. S. AGARWAL

SRI AUROBINDO ASHRAM
PONDICHERRY

First edition 1953
Fourth facsimile edition 1976
Eighth impression 2006

Price Rs 70
ISBN-10: 81-7058-068-4
ISBN-13: 978-81-7058-068-3

Published by Sri Aurobindo Ashram Publication Department
Pondicherry 605 002
Web: http://sabda.sriaurobindoashram.org

Printed at Sri Aurobindo Ashram Press, Pondicherry
PRINTED IN INDIA

# CONTENTS

# SECRETS OF INDIAN MEDICINE

## INTRODUCTION

HISTORY tells us about the supremacy of Indian culture and medicine in olden days. Evidently the consciousness of Indians of that time must have been more developed than that of other nations. What made those people great in their thoughts and actions? Persons who really discovered something for the good of humanity were the seers, thinkers and men of action. They had creative genius. Their intuitive faculty was highly developed. Their motive of life was the service of God through humanity. On such a sound basis they dared to achieve the highest truths in various aspects of life as well as of medicine.

Today the ancient medicine is in a deplorable condition because its followers have forgotten the spiritual idealism and intuitive faculty and are under the influence of materialistic ideas. The result is that spiritually they have become stagnant and have lost the creative genius. They have lost the true interpretation and application of Ayurvedic principles; hence there is downfall, and this profound, simple system of medicine has become very confusing to the modern mind.

The past knowledge is both a drag and a force for progress. It is the past that has created the present and a great part of it is creating the future. Modern medicine is the development of the ancient medicine. Both Allopathy and Ayurveda are working on the same lines. Ayurveda has given the general outlines of medicine while modern medicine has detailed each part of it with the help of highly developed intellect. We must take full account of the potent revelations of Allopathy and combine them with the luminous secrets of Ayurveda which seem to be veiled. The modern doctor will still find something simple and efficacious in Ayurveda and will be surprised to discover rare secrets worth applying to patients.

Being an Allopath myself my studies of Ayurvedic literature are limited and whatever I have learnt about Ayurveda is mostly a spontaneous growth which is mainly due to the divine grace. Opportunities came and the problems arose and I had to discover the solution. The first problem was put before me by a minister to write a paper on 'Synthetic Research in Ophthalmology'. The second problem arose after a lapse of two years when the editor of an Ayurvedic Journal wanted me to write some articles and I decided to elaborate the Tridosha theory. Again after a lapse of two years another problem arose and I was asked to write on the ancient methods of investigation to determine the qualities and actions of a drug.

If the Indian medicine is to accomplish its real mission it must start a double movement of revival and reform. It must revive its Tridosha theory on which the whole ancient medicine is based, so that it may appeal to the modern mind, and on the basis of this theory modify and purify its forms of application. These forms of medicine and modes of application must be simple and scientific to reveal the spirit of ancient medicine.

Ayurveda affirms that along with the gross material body there is a subtle body also which is quite plastic and mobile, not rigid like the material body. One feels the presence of this subtle body usually in the subconscient state, that is, during sleep in dreams when one finds oneself away from the body moving amongst different persons and at different places. To deal with the diseases of man efficiently the knowledge of both the gross material body and the subtle body is essential.

Ayurveda believes that like all other things man is also composed of five elements—earth, water, fire, air and ether. It is quite simple to understand; one eats food, drinks water, enjoys the sun, breathes the air and is alive due to the presence of ether or life-force. This life-force is the basis for man's mental and spiritual activities so that Nature may evolve him towards perfection. The function of each element is different. The earth gives shape to the body and releases its energy; bones, muscles and tissues represent it in the body without which no such shape of man would have been possible. Water makes the earth supple and helps in the transmission of energy; serum and lymph represent it, without which the body would have become a dry and rigid mass. Fire makes the form of the body steady and gives vigour and stimulation; digestion and circulation represent it. Air ignites the fire and works as a life carrier and is the support of all contact and exchange; respiration and the nervous system represent it. Ether is the creator of life itself in the body. A harmonious combination and function of these five elements produce a healthy and beautiful body.

In man both the lower and the higher Natures are present. The lower Nature expresses itself through lethargy, depression, disease, jealousy, hatred, anger, desire, passions, selfishness, doubts, wrong thinking etc., while the higher Nature expresses itself through love, kindness, courage, reason, benevolence, aspiration etc. The health of man is frequently influenced by the activities of these two different Natures and the aim of life is to transform the lower Nature and elevate it to the higher so that man may enjoy perfect health and happiness.

It is important to mention here that the pioneers of Ayurveda display some peculiarity in their expression. Their formula of speech is brief and adequate. It conceals the idea contained in their formulae from an average intelligence. There is multi-significance of each term—Vata, Pitta, Kapha—

in order to pack as much meaning as possible into a single word. This makes it very difficult to understand it at first sight. For example, Pitta means gastric juice, bile, energy, heat, inflammation, anger, irritation, etc.

Another remarkable feature of the early history of Ayurveda is that at first it expresses a small stock of ideas of Vata, Pitta and Kapha as humors. Afterwards there is a gradual increase in variety of idea and precision of idea. The progression is from the general to the particular, from the vague to the precise. The progression is worked out by processes of association of ideas. This is how Ayurveda describes disorders and treatment in a general and particular way in the symbolic terms like Vata, Pitta and Kapha.

When in modern speech we use the word 'saliva', we mean in the English language 'the secretion of salivary glands in the mouth,' but for the Acharyas 'Kapha' meant feeling of cold, heaviness, running of the nose, passing of mucoid discharge and also the saliva. Similarly Vayu meant mind, dryness, pain, flatulence, sensitiveness, lightness and also air. As the modern speech is quite different from the ancient, we shall endeavour to express the ancient compact ideas of medicine according to the present way of understanding through a series of articles published in this book. I hope these articles will prove a valuable key to the understanding of the ancient Indian medical literature. To illustrate the subject I shall frequently refer to the eye due to my familiarity with Ophthalmic science, but the principles are applicable to the diseases of other parts of the body as well.

Along with the evolution of man's intelligence, medicine has also evolved. At first the means of its evolution were sense faculties and intuition and that discovery of medicine was called Ayurveda. Then the intellect discovered various diagnostic instruments, such as the microscope, X'rays, Ophthalmoscope, etc., since the knowledge through sense perception was found insufficient by the rational mind; this discovery of medicine was called Allopathy. Hahnemann observed that the life-force was affected in sickness and he evolved Homeopathy. Bates noted that the mind came under a great strain in many diseases of the eye and body, and developed relaxation methods. Thus each system covers a part of the complex medicine and attempts to bring out its highest possibilities. A synthesis of all of them largely conceived and applied might well result in the integral system of medicine. But they are so disparate in their tendencies that we do not easily find how we can arrive at their right union. An undiscriminating combination will create confusion. The synthesis we propose must seize some central principle common to all which will include and utilize in the right place and proportion their particular principle. This book does not go into details of the particular principles of each system but gives an idea of the central principle of synthesis and the subject needs further investigation.

The central idea is that it is the Nature or Energy which heals a sick. This energy is either weak, dormant or perverted in a disease and a physician by his knowledge of medicine tries to awaken and properly adjust this energy of healing in his patient. We may say, "Then where is the necessity of a physician?" Yes, many people resist to any kind of treatment and get well; while many others go under rigid discipline of treatment and become worse. Every physician experiences such things in his practice. Yet, if a physician has a command over the handling of this natural energy he will be called a saviour; and this means he ought to have proper understanding of complex man, his nature and the forces that drive man's nature. Hence to become an efficient doctor the integral knowledge of man and medicine is essential but the proper sense of integration and efficiency will develop in a physician more and more by the evolution of spiritual knowledge.

We aim to create a new type of doctor whose guiding principle will be intuition, whose knowledge will be based on the synthesis, who will be more concerned with the health than with the pathology. Such a spiritualised doctor of the future will prove to be a physician *par excellence*, integrating all the systems of medicine harmoniously. In the diagnosis and treatment of patients he will be mainly guided by his intuition though he may also make use of modern scientific instruments to express the phenomena in scientific terms. In the treatment too he will mainly use his thought force and spiritual power, with or without medicines. His methods of treatment will be simple and harmless and will bring quick recovery, even in many so called hopeless cases. His very presence will radiate peace and healing force and his patient will be conscious of him as his saviour. He will create means which will bring health and happiness to suffering humanity as he himself will be hale and hearty, free from old age, incapacity and decay. To this physician of tomorrow this book is dedicated.

Dr. R. S. Agarwal

# CHAPTER I

## WHAT IS MAN?

MAN is a product of Nature. Everything including man has had a common origin in matter. Life manifested in matter, and Mind appeared in Life in the course of evolution. Man harbours within himself the Divine; without, he embraces the world. The Soul resides in the flesh and acts as a physician who knows and understands the disease of his patient but is not touched by the disease. The soul is also a link between man's past life and future life.

We observe that man develops three distinct personalities—the Mind, the Vital or Life, the Body. Through the mind he thinks and wills, through the vital he executes his thought and will, through the physical or body he expresses what he thinks or wills. A patient complained of blindness in his right eye and on examination the doctor came to the conclusion that the eye had cataract and decided to operate. On the day of the operation the doctor invoked the force to perform the operation through his hands and instruments, and the operation was very successful. The doctor's conclusion and decision was his mind, the force was his vital, the performance his body. The harmony between the mind, the vital and the body made the operation successful.

### Man's Nature or Gunas

These three parts of man—mind, vital and body—have different natures or gunas, called Sattwa, Rajas and Tamas.

1. Sattwa means principle of knowledge and harmony in

nature. This quality is represented by the mind.

2. Rajas—This principle in nature is characterised by desire, action and passion. The vital represents this quality.

3. Tamas—This is the principle of obscurity and inertia in nature and is represented by body.

Mind and vital are hidden in the body and evolve gradually. Take the example of a tiny baby, there is a little development of life but the mind is quite dormant. Gradually the life evolves and the child becomes active and naughty. As his development progresses desires, sex and passions also develop, and he tries for name and fame. This indicates how Rajas gradually grows in the child's body. When the child appears in the form of a man, he develops thinking power and reason and develops Sattwic character in himself.

## Action of Gunas in Man

So the man has three natures in himself—Sattwa, Rajas and Tamas. Man is driven by the forces of his Nature. Whatever desire comes, he tries to fulfil it; whatever emotion comes, he allows it to play; whatever physical wants he has, he tries to satisfy. This indicates that the activities and feelings of man are controlled by his Prakriti and mostly by the vital and physical nature. The body is the instrument of Prakriti or Nature—it obeys its own nature or it obeys the vital forces of desire, passion etc. But man has a mind and as he develops, he learns to control his vital and physical nature by his reason and by his will. This control is very partial; for the reason is often deluded by vital desires and the Tamas of the physical. Even if the reason keeps free and tells the vital or the body, "Do not do this" yet the vital and the body often follow their own movement in spite of the prohibition. This leads to suffering and disease.

## Physical Body

Man has gross physical body and subtle physical body. Man's gross physical and engine are similar in many respects. Both are made of matter (earth) and use plant products containing carbon for fuel (fire). They consume the fuel through the addition of inhaled oxygen (air) and exhale carbon dioxide produced during this process. They employ water which circulates through blood vessels and lymph vessels of the body and through the pipes of the machine as a heat conductor. The non-combustible residue is eliminated as ashes or faeces. Both transform the energy thus obtained into the motion of levers and joints. The Life-force runs the man, and man's force runs the machine.

Modern medicine has detailed the anatomy and physiology of the gross physical body which is visible to the external eye and on this subject the book "Secrets of Life" is sufficient for the beginners. The Subtle Physical Body is immediately behind the gross physical body and is closely connected with it. It has its subtle nervous system, centres of action and sense organs which correspond to the nervous system, ganglions and sense organs of the gross physical. The life-force which is different from material energy derived from food, pervades the gross physical through the subtle physical. The physician and physiologist are unaware of this life-force and subtle nervous system because they are not visible to the external sense organs but they can be vividly seen and experienced through intuition and inner vision. This life-force is the dynamic power of the human body and forms a subtle vital envelope around the gross physical. An infection attacking an individual should first pierce this subtle envelope which is quite weak ordinarily but by Yogic power and supramental force this can be greatly strengthened to defend all kinds of infections and adverse forces. In sickness and disturbed mental conditions the life-force is primarily affected and the function of different organs is disturbed.

## Two Kinds of Eyes in Man

The man has two kinds of eyes—one is external and the other is internal. The external eye is in flesh to see the outside world, while the inner eye belongs to the subtle body and is meant for the knowledge of invisible forces.

There are two external eyes and the act of seeing is passive. Things are seen just as they are felt or heard without effort. The eye with normal sight never makes an effort to see. The image received by the eye is transmitted to the visual centre in the hind part of the brain and the mind interprets this image. Therefore, the vision is a process of mental interpretation.

The inner eye has its seat between the two eye brows. In most men this eye is dormant but by voluntary will and Yogic practices this inner eye can develop. The function of the inner eye is to see invisible objects, actions and reactions of forces. What the inner eye sees is interpreted by the mind. The inner eye helps to have the true knowledge about a thing, action or thought while the external eye helps to the scientific approach. The vision of the inner eye is as vivid as the vision of the external eye. By the development of the inner eye intuition develops, and this faculty is a very valuable instrument to the external eye in the perfection of the body, works and researches.

Rishis who discovered Indian Medicine had developed the inner eye which revealed to them great truths about human life, vegetation and medicine. Rishi Dhanwantri has written qualities and actions of numerous herbs. At that time there was no laboratory, then how did he write them? Whatever he has written is mostly through his intuition. When he wanted to know the particulars of a certain herb, he sprinkled water on it with some mantra. The plant soon revealed its qualities and actions to the inner eye of the Rishi.

### Faculties of Man

Man has five faculties:

1. PHYSICAL FACULTY: There are five physical sense organs—eye to see, ear to hear, nose to smell, tongue to taste and skin to touch—through which man perceives objects. If any sense organ is damaged, its sense perception is automatically damaged. For example, a man becomes blind due to cataract, the faculty of seeing objects is automatically lost.

2. SUBTLE PHYSICAL FACULTY: There is a subtle faculty in man which can see, hear or smell at a distance far beyond what is normal to the physical sense organ. This subtle sense is very prominent in animals. Give a kerchief used by a man to a dog, it will spot the man amongst a thousand. An elephant will take you straight to a place miles away where there is water, if you are stranded in waterless surroundings. Where there is no question of sight or smell, even then the animals perceive things in a queer way: an elephant, again, for example, refusing to advance further upon road, because, as it was discovered later on, the road was hollow inside and would have sunk down had the animal walked upon it. There are other countless phenomena to prove the faculty of the animal sense or instinct as it is called. This subtle sense is greatly diminished in man due to the development of the

mind, but by training one can develop it to an extraordinary degree. For example, there was a person who could see physical objects, read and write, drive a car when the eye was perfectly bandaged.

3. VITAL FACULTY: Man has desires and passions and wants to progress in life; performs actions, also quarrels and fights. What drives him to do all this? This is the vital faculty in him.

4. MENTAL FACULTY: Man also thinks, forms ideas, makes schemes, reasons and criticises. What is it that enables him to do all that? This is his mental faculty.

5. PSYCHIC FACULTY: Man has a soul in him though many are unconscious of it. Due to the presence of the soul, the purest element in him, he loves beauty and art, aspires for peace and harmony, expresses kindness and love. This fine faculty in him is termed Psychic faculty. Persons in whom this faculty is developed participate in a higher and vaster life and do great works for the good of humanity.

## CHAPTER II

## Tridosha Philosophy of Ayurveda

### Tridhatu-Tridosha

THE Acharyas have put the whole philosophy of medicine in one word Tridhatu-Tridosha. 'Tri' means three principles—Vata, Pitta, Kapha—which have been freely used to simplify the medical science. In modern terms Vata may be called Mental, Pitta stands for Vital and Kapha for Physical. Vata, Pitta, Kapha are merely symbolic words and a symbol has a different meaning at each place of reference. For example, take the word 'Fire'. In material sense one sees fire in the burning wood, but fire will have a different meaning when the patient complains of fire burning in the body and this will mean that he has high temperature or great restlessness due to heat. Similarly when the patient complains of the fire of appetite, this means he is very hungry. Or when one remarks that his eyes are like fire, this means there is redness in the eyes. Thus at each place of reference the interpretation of 'fire' is different though linked with the symbol. Similarly Vata, Pitta, Kapha are symbolic terms used in medicine at different references and a correct and wide application of these principles is the key of success.

When the expression of Vata, Pitta, Kapha is about the health of man, the philosophy is termed as 'Tridhatu'; but when the expression is about disorders, the philosophy is termed as 'Tridosha'. The whole conception is so simple, scientific and artistic that the intellect finds difficulty in the correct interpretation of Vata, Pitta and Kapha but a true grasp of the subject makes the various aspects of medicine easy to understand and expressible in terms of modern medicine so called Allopathy. The following are some illustrations about 'Tridhatu-Tridosha'.

## Tridhatu

For the existence of life and health man eats food, enjoys sun and breathes air. Here air is for Vata, sun for Pitta and food for Kapha.

What he eats and drinks is digested with the help of air which he breathes, gastric juice and saliva. Here air is Vata, gastric juice is Pitta and saliva is Kapha.

Out of what he eats, a portion is absorbed, mixed in blood for circulation in the system for the formation of various cells of the body. In each cell the nucleus is for Vata, protoplasm for Pitta, and cell's body for Kapha.

Various cells develop bones and muscles, blood, brain and nervous system which have three distinct functions. Here Brain or thinking motor or mind stands for Vata.

Blood or vitality or vital stands for Pitta.

Bones and muscles or body stands for Kapha.

The harmonious action of mind, vital and body produces health. For the harmonious action of the mind man needs rest and relaxation; for the vital he needs control over palate, sex and desires; for the body he requires physical exercise, proper diet and formation of healthy physical habits. Out of what man eats, drinks or inhales, a portion is passed out of the body as excretion. Here exhaled air is for Vata, urine and perspiration for Pitta, faeces for Kapha.

## Tridosha

The following are some illustrations about the application of the three principles when the health of man is affected.

1. *Expulsion of Dosha in material form:* Here mucoid discharge through the nose, mouth, anus, eye etc. is Kapha; yellow or watery discharge as in vomiting, urine, watering of eye etc. is called Pitta; belching or any other manifestation of wind is called Vata; passing of pus as in rhinitis, gonorrhoea, abscess etc. is called Tridosha.

2. *Feeling of dosha in the body:* Feeling of cold is kapha; feeling of heat is Pitta; feeling of pain and dryness is Vata; and feeling of unusual symptoms as in delirium, floating specks etc. is called Tridosha.

3. *Cause of diseases:* A disharmony between the mind, the vital and the body or so to say between Vata, Pitta and Kapha can be found as the cause of most of the illnesses and diseases. Usually the primary cause is accumulation of toxic matter (Kapha), or lack of vitality (Pitta), or lack of relaxation (Vata) in the body.

The secondary causes like infection, fear, irregularities in diet and habits, atmospheric conditions etc. are able to attack the man when the primary cause is present.

Three humors—air, gastric juice and saliva—constantly circulate in the body and help in digestion and health. When their equilibrium is disturbed due to any reason, the digestion and health of the body or of any particular organ are impaired.

4. *Classification of diseases:* Here the interpretation is rather different. Here Vata is for painful or paralytic diseases as neuralgia, paralysis etc., Pitta is for inflammatory diseases as fevers, iritis, redness, conjunctivitis etc. Kapha is for non-inflammatory diseases as simple glaucoma etc. Tridosha

is for prulent and degenerative diseases as abscess, coma, ne-
phritis, staphyloma etc. A disease may pass through one or
more or all the stages or may be a combination of two or three
stages. For example, there is some discomfort at a localised
place on the thumb without any sign of inflammation, this is
the Kaphaja stage. The discomfort turns into a red pimple
showing signs of inflammation, now this is the Pittaja stage.
The pimple becomes very painful and this is the Vataja stage.
Then pus forms in it and this is the Tridosha stage.

Another example, a patient has redness in the eyes accompanied by pain and mucoid discharge, such a disease can be
classified as Vataja due to the presence of pain, as Pittaja due
to redness, and as Kaphaja due to presence of mucoid discharge, but cannot be called Tridosha as there is no degeneration.

Or a patient is suffering from chronic dacryocystitis, a
condition in which pus flows out from the side of the nose
into the eye. There is no pain or any inflammation. Such a
disease is classified as Tridosha.

5. *Treatment:* In treatment also three main principles have
been applied:

(a) Elimination (Kapha): Elimination of unwanted or toxic
matter which may be done through purgatives, enemas, emetics, diuretics, diaphoretics, errhines, operations, antitoxic
drugs and injections, irritating medicines; elimination of
wrong habits etc.

(b) Stimulation (Pitta): Stimulation means to improve
blood circulation, immunity and vitality which may be
achieved through deep breathing, exercise, vapour bath, sun
bath, tonics, vitamins, diet, digestives, massage, invigorating
medicines, injections, drawing energy from the Universe,
Homeopathy etc.

(c) Relaxation (Vata): Relaxation of mind and nerves may be produced by autosuggestion, faith cure, concentration, meditation, relaxation exercises, rest, right use of the organs, hygienic and pleasant surroundings, fasting, soothing medicines, analgesics, hypnotics, narcotics etc.

## Different Types and Forms of Vata, Pitta and Kapha

Here the description is anatomical and physiological and each has been described in five forms with five functions.

*Five forms of Vata:* These are the five main centres of the subtle physical body and correspond to the nervous plexuses.

1. Material or Muladhar centre (Apan): This centre corresponds to the pelvic plexus and is the seat of Kundalini or material energy and controls excretions.

2. Naval centre (Saman): This corresponds to the Solar plexus in the naval region and controls digestion.

3. Heart centre (Prana)—refers to the Cardiac plexus in the heart region and controls heart and circulation.

4. Throat centre (Udan)—corresponds to the Pharyngeal plexus, in the throat region and controls breathing and speech.

5. Forehead centre (Vyan)—corresponds to the Nasociliary plexus at the root of the nose and base of the skull and controls Will.

*Five forms of Pitta:*

1. Gastric juice which gives appetite and helps digestion.
2. Bile which gives complexion to the skin.
3. Haemoglobin which colours the blood.
4. Aquous Humor which brightens the eyes.

5. Life energy which controls the whole body.

*Five forms of Kapha:*

1. Saliva which helps mastication.
2. Cerebrospinal fluid which keeps the head cool.
3. Lymph which gives taste.
4. Serum which helps the heart in pumping.
5. Synovial fluid which lubricates and aids free movements of the joints.

CHAPTER III

# HUMORS OF THE BODY

CHARAKA and Sushruta Samhitas are supposed to be the authority on Ayurveda. There are many interpreters who have written the translation and comments in various languages. Most of the writers seem to be confused in the explanation of the basic principles and the philosophy of Ayurveda. The basic principles Vata, Pitta and Kapha, on which the whole philosophy of medicine is based, are simply symbolic terms. When one discovers the true sense of these symbolic terms, one is simply surprised about the profound expression and the genius of the Rishis.

Today with the development of sharp intellect medicine has much advanced. What was impossible for the senses, has been discovered through intelligent and scientific means. With the aid of microscope the life of a cell and bacteria has been revealed. Under the microscope milk is not simply a white fluid but reveals millions of silvery fat globules and protein particles contained in it.

There are three humors—Vata, Pitta and Kapha—which are absorbed and circulated in the body having some definite qualities. But what are they actually?

1. VATA is dry, cold, subtle, rough, unstable and light. This humor is AIR we inhale, which is constantly in circulation with the blood in the system. It has all the above qualities. How?

Dry—expose a wet cloth to the air and it is dried.

Cold—expose a cup of hot tea to the air and it becomes cold.

Subtle—You don't see air but feel.

Rough—Skin exposed to air appears rough when there is no moisture.

Unstable—because air freely moves.

Light—because it goes up from the ground.

2. PITTA is hot, acid, mobile, liquid, acute and pungent. This humor is GASTRIC JUICE which is absorbed in the system and it has all the above qualities. How?

Hydrochloric acid is the main constituent of gastric juice. Take a bottle of hydrochloric acid and test its qualities. It is hot on touch, acid in reaction. It is liquid and mobile. But if you can just put a drop on the skin, you will find it acute and irritant. But when you taste dilute hydrochloric acid, it is pungent.

3. KAPHA is cold, heavy, immobile, sweet, soft, unctuous and viscid. All these qualities are found in SALIVA which is constantly secreted by salivary glands and is absorbed in the system with or without food. On touch you will find that saliva is cold, soft and viscid. If you spit on the ground, it remains steady. It gives sweet taste when you eat a piece of bread. When you rub it on the skin it gives unctuous complexion.

The three humors—air, gastric juice and saliva—circulate in the system in different proportions, help in digestion of food and general make up of the body. Though each of them has a different function, yet it is harmony, the right proportion of each, the proper combination of the three humors which is responsible for good health and good digestion. Their harmony can be maintained to a great extent by exercise, regulation of diet, adoption of natural urges as urine, faeces, flatus, thirst, hunger etc., proper use of senses and desires and good thinking.

## Composition and Function of Humors

1. AIR—Air is essential for keeping up the vibration of life, respiration, oxidation and combustion, circulation of blood, regular elimination of stools, urine, perspiration and carbon-dioxide.

The air is a mixture of various gases consisting of about 79% of nitrogen, 20 per cent oxygen and one per cent other gases. Nitrogen helps in building protoplasm while oxygen is chemically very active in the process of oxidation as it smashes a molecule and combines with its fragments. Cut an apple in two pieces and observe the cut surface. After a while it turns brown because the oxygen of the air acts upon the exposed molecules and breaks them up into simpler compounds possessing a brown colour. In the course of oxiding process the atoms acted upon vibrate and emit energy waves which impinge upon our senses as heat. An oxiding process characterised by the development of light and heat is known as combustion.

Fire is produced by the union of oxygen atoms with the molecules of a fuel substance. Man takes oxygen and fuel substances as food into his body where oxidation takes place, producing heat. This heat makes human life possible. The intake of oxygen is called respiration. The human body is warm because oxidation and combustion are present in it; and this process takes place because it breathes. A breathing human being is a continuous furnace in which the carbon of ingested food is slowly and uninterruptedly consumed throughout life by the oxygen of the inspired air at a constant temperature of 98.6F.

2. GASTRIC JUICE—Gastric glands of the stomach secrete gastric juice which is responsible for digestion of food, heat in the body, complexion of the skin and lustre in the eyes.

The chief constituents of gastric juice are hydrochloric acid, pepsin and rennin.

Hydrochloric acid accelerates the action of pepsin and stimulates the muscle fibres of the stomach wall to promote digestion. It activates the digestive apparatus in the neighbouring sections of the intestinal tract. As soon as the stomach secretes hydrochloric acid, not only the stomach but also the duodenum begins to exhibit peristaltic waves, the liver secretes bile, and pancreas pancreatic juice. Hydrochloric acid is disinfectant also and there is no putrifaction in a healthy stomach. We ingest billions of bacilli daily with our food, yet they do not harm because they fall into a gigantic lake of hydrochloric acid and die there.

Pepsin is a ferment and helps in the digestion of protein; food that enters the stomach as protein leaves it through the pylorus after chemical change as peptone.

Rennin is also a ferment of gastric juice for the digestion of milk and splits the protein of milk into casein. When an infant vomits, it does not bring out milk, but casein. Rennin also attacks the fat of milk. If a person eats three different kinds of fat during a meal—for instance, olive oil in the salad, fish oil and butter—only the last named fat, since it is milk product, will be digested in the stomach. We are right in saying that fatty foods take longer to digest because stomach does not digest any fats except milk fat; other fats are digested in the lower sections of the intestine. Large quantities of fat slow down gastric digestion because the fat covers the other foods and renders it difficult for the gastric juice to come into contact with the food.

3. SALIVA is the secretion of the glands in the mouth. The parotid is the largest gland and secretes large quantities of watery saliva. The glands near the lower jaw are smaller and

produce small quantities of mucus saliva. The watery saliva of the upper gland serves chiefly to dilute and moisten the food well; the mucus saliva renders the food slippery. Depending on the kind of food, the secretion of the one or the other gland predominates. If we bite a juicy apple that does not have to be moistened, the lower salivary glands secrete a scanty mucus saliva. On the other hand, if we eat a biscuit, the parotid begins to function, producing large quantities of watery saliva containing little mucus. The activity of salivary glands is excited by reflex means.

The human saliva contain water 99.4 per cent, salts, 0.2 per cent, mucus 0.2 per cent, ferment 0.2 per cent. The ferment contained in saliva is known as amylase because it breaks starch into malt sugar which tastes sweet. Put a piece of bread in your mouth and let it lie there. It does not change nor does it have any taste. When it is chewed thoroughly and mixed with saliva it becomes sweet. Being watery it is cooling and soothing; being salty, saliva is alkaline in reaction. Being mucoid it is viscid and unctuous.

# Chapter IV

# HUMORAL DISORDERS

Modern medical science recognises the great importance of air, gastric juice and saliva as humors in the process of digestion and metabolism etc. but does not express in terms of Vata, Pitta and Kapha. It explains all the qualities of air, gastric juice and saliva in a detailed scientific way and these qualities tally with the description of Vata, Pitta and Kapha as humors in the language of Ayurveda.

What man eats, drinks, or masticates, is digested with the action of saliva, gastric juice and air, but he does not live on what he eats but rather on what he digests. The body is not nourished by what we ingest, but by what passes from the intestine through the liver into the blood. The fluid that passes from the intestine into the blood is called 'nutrient fluid'. The quality of nutrient fluid depends on the quality of food. The various kinds of nourishment taken by man, on being well digested by various ferments and juices whose strength is kept active by the inner gastric juice (Pitta) circulate in the body.

The nutrient fluid mixed in the blood is taken to the whole body tissues where the cells transform the blood substance into energy, and thus the metabolic process of all the body elements goes on constantly. The cells reject what is not required and the rejected matter is thrown out of the body with faeces, urine, sweat, breath, excretions of eye, nose, ear, mouth, hair follicles and generative organs etc. The ultimate elements are absorbed and energy material is formed in the form of blood, tissues, flesh, fat, bone, marrow, semen and vital essence etc. In this way the essential and waste fluids retaining their proper proportions keep up the balance of the elements in the normally constituted body and the body enjoys health, vitality, complexion and cheerfulness.

Modern science is unable to explain how the inanimate substance, nutrient fluid, circulating in the blood is transformed into animate nature or living matter commonly called protoplasm which is a marvellous phenomenon of life.. According to Ayurveda there is life or consciousness in inanimate matter too which is hidden and involved in the matter. But when matter passes under a certain process, the hidden life appears as a living thing. It is why Ayurveda advises to offer the food to the Divine first and then eat: it means calling down the Divine influence on the food. If one knows how to do it, it would diminish very much the labour of the inner transformation i.e. change of inanimate substance into animate form.

Protoplasm is not a chemical compound but rather a complex organisation of life. In order to have some idea of the complicated structure of this living matter let us compare it with a watch. Place your watch before you and just think of the complexity of its mechanism. It consists of more than a hundred parts: screws, shafts, cog-wheels of various sizes, springs, hinges, levers, a dial and hands, all systematically and skilfully assembled in a working mechanism of the greatest precision. Now imagine this watch growing smaller before our eyes. Without losing any part of it or ceasing to function, it becomes as small as a rice grain or a sugar granule, and finally it disappears. If we now take a microscope and look for the watch at the spot where it vanished, we rediscover it with all its parts intact and functioning. Such is the picture which we should have in mind when we think of protoplasm.

HUMORAL DISORDERS: When for some reason as lack of

exercise or over exercise, irregularities of dietetic rules, suppression of urges (passing of wind, stools, urine, vomiting etc.) seasonal abnormality, desires and passion, fear, worries, wrong thinking etc., the humors are disturbed, bodily disorders take place. For example, feeling of dryness in the throat, heat and irritation in the eyes, cold and heaviness in the head. Dryness is the quality of air (Vata), heat and irritation are the qualities of gastric juice (pitta), cold and heaviness are the qualities of saliva (Kapha). That is why when such a disorder takes place, it is termed as provoked Vata or Pitta or Kapha. Now the question is from where these symptoms of dryness, heat and cold arose? The elements of air, gastric juice and saliva are circulating in the tissues of the body through blood and the above symptoms are the qualities of these humors. Therefore, when one or more humors are provoked, their qualities appear as a disturbance in the form of dryness, heat or cold. Such symptoms may appear in the whole body or in any part of the body. It is specially in this type of disorders that Ayurveda plays an important role in the treatment and maintains superiority over all other systems.

TREATMENT OF HUMORAL DISORDERS: When the symptoms of dryness, heat or cold are prominent Ayurveda suggests two methods to determine the lines of treatment.

1. FIRST METHOD: According to the first method prescribe the opposite in action, that is, if the symptom of heat is present, prescribe cold things; and in case of dryness, unctuous substances, while in case of cold give hot things. On this basis Ayurveda gives a long list of articles but I mention here only a few.

For dryness (Vata)—Clarified butter, oil, fat, bone-marrow, milk etc.

For heat (Pitta)—cold water, wet mud plaster, white of egg,

curd, corriander, sandal, rose, brahmi etc.

For cold (Kapha)—Hot water, honey, ginger, asafoetida, Kasturi etc.

2. SECOND METHOD: According to the second method prescription will depend on the taste of things, as different tastes relieve dryness, heat or cold. There are six important tastes—sweet, sour, alkaline, astringent, bitter and pungent.

DRYNESS (Vata)—Sweet, sour and alkaline tastes subdue dryness while pungent, bitter and astringent tastes increase dryness. For example, during the hot and dry weather when there is a feeling of dryness in the body, a glass of syrup or lemon juice mixed with water and sugar or a cup of salt water or raw mango boiled and mixed with salt, sugar and water, relieves the condition of dryness quickly. But the prescription of ginger, karela (bitter gourd) and articles which have pungent, astringent and bitter tastes will aggravate the feeling of dryness.

HEAT (Pitta)—Sweet, astringent and bitter tastes relieve the symptoms of heat and its discomforts, while sour, pungent and alkaline tastes aggravate the trouble. For example, when there is a feeling of heat in the body, a glass of syrup will quickly refresh the system. Or when the feeling of heat and discomfort is due to secretion of increased gastric juice, the various sweet preparations will satisfy the hunger but prescription of lemon, chillies and salty articles will aggravate the trouble. When the heat is accompanied with inflammation, neem, chirata, herar (terminelia chebula), rasot which are astringent and bitter help in reducing the inflammatory condition.

COLD (Kapha)—Pungent, astringent and bitter tastes relieve cold while sweet, sour and salt tastes increase the trouble. For example, when there is a feeling of cold, pepper, ginger, cloves, onion, karela help to relieve the coldness but eating sweetmeats and sour raw mangoes will aggravate the trouble.

INTERESTING CASES: 1. A man aged about thirty years with high myopia was suffering from insomnia for several months. He was feeling heat and burning sensation as if fire was coming out of his hands and feet. Various medicines prescribed by doctors could not induce sleep except for an hour or so in the beginning only. He then applied mud soaked in cold water on cloth pieces and put them on hands and feet at bed time. From that very day he began to have good sleep and he repeated this process for several months. In the morning he was finding the mud plaster quite hot. Mud has the quality of retaining the cold or heat for a long time.

2. A girl patient after a short illness developed severe headache. She had a feeling of dryness in the eyes, nose and ears. Her digestion was very good. When the modern doctors failed to relieve headache, she consulted a Kaviraj who advised the girl to take varieties of food containing sufficient clarified butter and sugar. The girl preferred 'halwa' or 'Upma', a preparation of wheat flour, ghee and sugar. Side by side the physician prescribed dropping of sweet oil in the nose and ears and application of butter in the eyes at bed time, also massage of head with 'brahmi oil'. The result was the patient was cured in a few days and improved her health considerably. The chief thing in this case was that the nervous tissue was in great need of fatty nourishment and due to lack of such nourishment the patient was getting the symptoms of dryness and headache.

3. A patient was suffering from severe headache on one side of the head from sunrise to sunset. There was a feeling of cold and heaviness in the head. At times the discomfort was so great that he liked to dash his head against a wall. He was

prescribed dry ginger powder mixed in milk to drop in the nostrils before sunrise. This created irritation in the nose and throat and much mucus began to flow out and the patient was completely cured. There are various medicines of this type which can be safely used as mild errhines or strong errhines. Modern medicine is yet far behind to tackle such diseases successfully.

4. In another case there was persistent redness in the eyes without discharge. The feeling of heat was prominent. The doctors were treating the patient with various medicines commonly used for trachoma and the trouble had aggravated due to irritating medicines. However, this patient was cured by the use of rose water and sandal paste around the eyes. He was given Triphala at bed time and was advised to avoid pungent and bitter things as pickles, chillies, karela.

5. A patient was using glasses for several years. His eyes looked dull, lusterless and wrinkled. At times he felt some discomfort in the eyes. The patient was given a course of Tarpana treatment as Ayurveda has prescribed to brighten the eyes. Tarpana is a sort of eye wash with clarified butter mixed with warm water. The result was that his eyes became bright, full of life though defective vision continued. Has modern science discovered any such process which can brighten the eyes, develop 'tejas' in them?

6. An eminent doctor's mother was having great itching sensation at the lid margins of both the eyes and she rubbed the lids at times so much that scratches formed. This constant itching sensation became a troublesome affair and she had to remove her glasses so as to rub the lids frequently. The doctors had prescribed various eye drops and eye ointments to apply in the eyes, but somehow missed the idea of advising the patient to apply and rub the ointment on the lids and lid

margins. However, her itching sensation was completely relieved in a week's time by applying milk cream on the eyelids at bed time. This itching sensation was due to dryness, due to lack of fatty element in the tissues, especially at the root of eye lashes. Later on the patient told me that she applied sufficient quantity of hair oil on the head and it was quickly absorbed.

VITIATED CONDITION OF HUMORS: When there is putrifaction in the stomach or intestine it gives rise to unaggreeable symptoms as erructations, flatulence, colic etc., and the main seat of accumulation of gases (Vata) is the large intestine and enema is the quick process to relieve such conditions. Ayurveda gives a long list of various types of enemas.

When gastric juice (pitta) is vitiated in the digestive canal, it accumulates in the vitiated condition in the small intestine and one may get fever, inflammation, indigestion etc., and purgative is the quickest process to relieve the disorder. There is a long list of purgatives for selection.

When saliva (Kapha) is vitiated in the digestive system, its chief seat of accumulation is stomach and one feels loss of appetite, disinclination for sweet and rich food, sweet taste, nausesa and vomiting; and emetics bring quick relief in such disorders. There are various emetics, some are mild while others are strong.

Humoral disorder is a frequent happening in the human being, hence most people suffer from digestive disorders. These disorders when neglected or not properly treated give rise to many diseases of liver and circulation, diseases of respiratory system, urinary system, nervous system etc. and may even lead to serious complications.

# Chapter V

# EFFECT OF CONSTITUTIONAL DISORDERS
## ON EYE AND BODY

USUALLY in the treatment of a particular disease of an organ as conjunctivitis, glaucoma, headache etc., the older Acharyas laid great stress on the constitution of the patient. Within certain limits they were doubtless right. Treatment based on their knowledge and experience can cure many so called incurable cases. Today their important studies on the constitutional factor in diseases are almost forgotten by the present generation. It is true former ideas require much revision in the light of modern research, but that does not imply that all the teaching of our medical forefathers ought to be discarded. Too much attention is now being paid to the germ and too little to the soil on which it grows. This is a matter for regret. Laboratory knowledge is most helpful and invaluable so far as it goes, but real experience in the diagnosis and treatment of the disease must be gained in the clinic. What are designated "Scientific methods" practised in laboratories are threatening to displace the art and science of healing. Disease reveals itself by its symptoms and the earliest signs are manifested by sensations and feelings of the sick man himself. These symptoms cannot, however, be analysed in a test-tube. A very short clinical experience will prove that micro-organisms do not always behave in the same manner, especially in human beings; their actions vary according to the vitality of the patient. Hence the study of constitutional disorders is necessary to relieve the human sufferings.

To deal with the constitutional disorders Ayurveda gives

the formula in a nutshell in its language of Vata, Pitta, Kapha. Mostly when there is a disorder three factors are present:

1. Accumulation of toxic matter (Kapha)
2. Lack of vitality and energy (Pitta)
3. Lack of rest and relaxation (Vata)

ACCUMULATION OF TOXIC MATTER: (Kapha) In the act of living there is a constant manufacture of toxic products which are mostly removed through faeces and urine, also through perspiration, exhaled air and discharges of mouth and nose. But in most cases when intake of proteins, fats and sugar is greater than what can be assimilated, the eliminative activity is retarded, the digestion is disturbed, the liver becomes sluggish, the function of the kidneys becomes inadequate. The waste products are accumulated in the body, thereby causing derangement of health. Usually there is complaint of constipation or the motions are unnatural in quantity, colour and smell. Flatulence is often present. Deposits in urine are often found. In short when the toxic matter is absorbed in the blood the patient is vulnerable to every form of infection. Hence nutritional defects causing the accumulation of toxic matter are the primary cause of many diseases as retinitis, acute conjunctivitis, iritis, acute glaucoma etc.

LACK OF VITALITY AND ENERGY: (Pitta) All the tissues of the body are bathed in lymph and each cell draws the nourishment from it and casts waste products into it. In health delicate physiological balance between assimilation and excretion takes place, and a breakdown in that arrangement is one of the earliest departures from health. When there is accumulation of toxic matter in the cells, the toxins enter into blood, the capillaries are distended and circulation of blood is affected. Consequently the functional activity of an organ or organs of the body is disturbed, especially the liver becomes sluggish,

and this leads to lack of vitality. The patient notices a difference and says "I am quite well but not feeling strong"or "I
take my food but I am never hungry". When there is lack of
vitality the resistence to outside influence is decreased. In
old age often people complain that the eyesight varies according
to the general health.

## How blood is vitiated according to Ayurveda:

1. By intoxicants, excessive use of alkaline, salty, sour,
pungent articles and excessive use of green vegetables.
2. Things which cause indigestion and constipation.
3. Mental disturbances.
4. Use of incompatible articles at a time.

LACK OF REST AND RELAXATION (Vata):

Muscle fibres are supplied by nerve endings. The toxin
circulating in the blood and reaching the muscles excites or
inhibits the terminations of nerves. This may happen in one
organ or in several organs of the body. If the effect is of excita-
tion of nerve endings, the result is pain and discomfort followed by congestion and inflammation. If the effect is of inhibi-
tion, then there is lethargy, laziness, heaviness, lack of activity
in the function of the organ. Consequently the mind gets
strain and the blood circulation in the brain is disturbed. The
mental control and thought are affected. When the mind is
under strain, the eye is also influenced when it makes an
effort to see. Not only the eye but all the vital processes of
digestion, assimilation, elimination get disturbed by mental
strain.

TREATMENT: The physician must know that the cause of a disease may not necessarily be found in the organ manifesting the symptoms, and that no treatment can be successful until the cause underlying the disease has been discovered and removed. In some cases, however, the disease may be due to some local structural and functional defect rather than a general constitutional weakness; in such cases the treatment may not replace the structutal defect but in majority of cases disordered functional defect can be restored. Ayurveda describes the treatment in its symbolic language.

1. ELIMINATION OF TOXIC MATTER (Kapba)

This may be achieved by purgatives, enemas, fast, diuretics, diaphoretics, emetics, errhines, operation, irritant medicines etc.

*Purgatives*: Triphala, senna, castor oil, rhubarb, Ispgol etc.

*Diuretics*: Sugar cane juice, fruit juice, barley water, soup, potassium nitrate etc.

*Diaphoretics*: Hot drinks, vapour bath, dry ginger powder with milk, Sanafsha decoction, black peper decoction, exercise etc.

*Emetics*: Drinking salt water, copper sulphate etc.

*Errhines*: Soapnut water, sharbindu oil, onion juice, ginger juice.

STIMULATION (Pitta) Stimulation means increasing the vitality by improving the quality, quantity and flow of blood. This process is usually adopted after elimination but some in cases its use is imminent. The following means are useful:

Massage, exercise, sun bath, hot bath, fomentation, infra-red therapy, tonics, liverextract, haemoglobin, digestives, cholagogues etc. Homeopathy to stimulate the dormant energy.

RELAXATION (Vata): Circulation of blood is very largely influenced ty rest and relaxation of the nerves and mind.

When the mind is under relaxation, that is, not attended by excitement or strain, the circulation in the brain is normal. The supply of blood to the eye and visual centre is normal and the vision is perfect. Not only the eye, but all the other sense organs and other vital organs receive good blood circulation. The cause of most eye troubles and other diseases of the body is abnormal thought which causes strain on the mind. We can consciously think thoughts which disturb the circulation and lower the visual power; we can also consciously think thoughts that will restore normal circulation. For example, there is a letter round 'O', imagine it in an abnormal way in the form of a square or triangle; observe that there is a feeling of discomfort and defective vision. Now imagine it round, in a normal way according to the reality without effort, and note the vision becomes clear and the head becomes light.

There are various methods to rest the mind and to improve its faculty as palming, imagination exercises, autosuggestion, inducing good sleep, soothing massage and soothing appplications etc.

Then there is a power within oneself which can develop the power of the mind, change the character of a person, control the functions of the body etc. ; and this power can be developed by meditation and concentration. Of course, one needs a spiritual teacher to learn such things.

A patient usually needs the application of all the three principles—elimination, stimulation and relaxation; but in some cases elimination may be the primary need while in others stimulation or relaxation may be of primary importance. To illustrate the subject I quote here a few cases.

CASE No. 1. Usually in the inflammatory conditions elimination is the primary method and relaxation follows it. A patient had an attack of inflammation of the eye, iritis. There was redness, watering, discomfort, photophobia. This patient had such attacks before also and each time took one or two months to recover. This time when the patient attended the clinic, a strong enema was given and sufficient mucus passed out with stools. Light diet without sweetmeats and milk preparations were given for a few days. Locally the eye was given gentle fomentation and bandaged after soothing drops. The patient was given complete rest. The result was that the attack subsided next day and the patient was perfectly all right within a week's time.

CASE No. 2. A child was gradually developing night blindness and his digestion was good. He was given Triphala Ghrita and Vitamin A preparations to nourish the cells of the eye. Locally he was advised to apply medicated honey in the eyes and then face the morning sun with eyes closed for a few minutes. The child got quick relief from night blindness. The diet contained more sugar, butter and milk. Every morning he was given fresh butter mixed with sugar and black pepper. Black pepper stimulates gastric fire while sugar helps digestion of fat. In this case the principle of stimulation was the primary need.

CASE No. 3. A patient aged about forty years was suffering from chronic retinitis (chronic inflammation of the retina) and eyesight was gradually failing. He usually remained constipated. His doctor had told him that it was not possible to improve the sight and that he may become blind after sometime. This increased his worry and he was quickly excited on petty matters.

There is a close relation between the mind and eyes and the body. In most cases it is the mind which makes the body or the eye suffer or at least it plays an important part in the illness. The mind possesses a certain power to act directly on the eye and the body in the formation of a disease, also in its cure.

This patient was advised to take the treatment on the lines of three principles in this order—relaxation, elimination and stimulation. When he was assured that he would improve his eyesight in a short time, he felt greatly relieved from his worry of losing eyesight. Then he was educated to relax his mind and eyes by relaxation exercises as palming, swinging. In palming he gently closed his eyes and covered them with the palms of his hands, avoiding any pressure on the eyeballs. When his eyes were closed and covered he counted 100 to 200 breathings to keep his mind concentrated. He repeated this process about 5 times a day. Also some medicines were applied in his eyes and the eyes were bandaged at times. The eyes and mind felt great comfort and the vision began to improve from the third day of the treatment.

For elimination he was given 'Triphala' or Ispgol' with milk at bed time. Once a week an enema was advised. Nasal drops of Sharbindu oil were used every morning for some days to bring out discharge through the nose. Also he eliminated his wrong habits of looking at things and replaced them by right habits as gentle blinking etc.

To adopt the principle of stimulation the patient faced the morning sun with closed eyes after the application of medicated honey in the eyes. Triphala ghirta, liver extract with vitamins were advised to be taken by mouth. Some eye exercises were practised on eye charts. The result was that the patient improved his vision considerably in a month's time.

*Case No.* 4. A lady patient was suffering from headache for fourteen days. The doctors were giving aspirin, bromides etc. to relieve her headache. In the beginning she had some relief but later on such drugs failed to give any relief and she developed insomnia. When I was called to treat this lady, I just observed her face which appeared to me under a great strain. So I gave her head massage with medicated oil for fourteen minutes and the headache was almost completely relieved and she could have a sound sleep. She was advised to practise palming several times a day and continue head massage morning and evening. The treatment in this case was mainly based on relaxation.

## Important Hints

1. A disease may first exist alone and later subside by giving rise to other diseases. For example, coryza may first appear and then may cause cough; cough causing wasting may cause consumption.

2. Treatment which cures the original disease but produces some other kind of complication, is not the correct line of treatment.

3. One cause may lead to many diseases or a single cause may lead to a single disease. Many causative factors may lead to many diseases. For example, constipation may cause fever, giddiness, headache, indigestion etc. or may cause only indigestion.

4. A single remedy may cure many diseases or there may be one remedy for one particular disesse. There may be many remedies for one disease or many diseases.

5. Light diet cures many gastrogenous diseases and fever.

6. An easily curable disease is cured by easy measures and in a short period, while formidable diseases are cured only by great efforts and after a long time.

Incurable diseases as absolute glaucoma or complete optic atrophy never become curable, while curable diseases may become incurable by improper treatment.

7. The wise physician should investigate the changes in the body elements, strength of the body, gastric fire, vitality and mind. Observe the variations in the disease and treat accordingly.

8. Morbid humors when they spread sideways from the alimentary canal and affect the urinary system or nervous system etc. afflict the patient for a long time. Under such conditions one should not be in a hurry to counteract the morbid humors. Morbid humors should be eliminated through a slow process or drawn painlessly into the alimentary canal and then removed.

9. Four factors are necessary in the successful treatment of bad cases.

a. Physician—He must have clear knowledge and mind and practical experience. His conduct towards the patient should be friendly and compassionate.

b. Drugs and therapeutic measures.

c. Nurse—A nurse must know the art of nursing and should have affection towards the sick.

d. Patient—obedience, courage, ability to describe himself are the signs of a good patient.

10. Specific diseases need specific treatment also but too much drugging, especially drastic ones, should always be avoided.

### Fatal Prognosis

Our medical forefathers could foretell the danger long before its coming by reading the face and mind of the patient. From whatever cause the death may arise, the early symptoms are sure to appear. Any sudden change in constitution or in senses usually indicates fatal prognosis. For example,

1. Abnormal discolouration of half or whole body without cause.

2. If half face dry and depressed and the other half animated.

3. If nose, eyes, ears and eyebrows are seen loose, out of position.

4. Tie a few hairs of head and pull. If they come out with roots without causing pain, the patient will die soon within six months.

5. Body exudes unpleasant smell and the patient has very sweet taste.

6. Those who are about to die perceive all things in their oppposite characteristics. For example, seeing invisible things or failing to see visible things.

7. Holds fingers in front of eyes and searches them.

8. Reflected image not visible in eye.

9. If disease leaves the weakened patient all of a sudden.

10. Ailing man that is afflicted at once with thirst, dyspnoea, headache and loose stools, gives up his life quickly.

11. If a man acquires or looses his robustness without any knowable cause and in an abnormal manner he dies within a year.

12. Formation of prominent network of vessels or crescent shaped furrows on forehead, which were not before, indicate death within six months.

13. Chest region dries up very soon after a bath while rest of the body remains wet, is an indication of fatal prognosis in a month's time.

CHAPTER VI

## FUNCTIONAL DISORDERS

AYURVEDA indicates that in the beginning when an organ does not function in a normal way, there is no sign of any organic change; the functional disorder can be easily cured in the early stage. Later on the functional disorder when not treated properly may become incurable or may become the cause of organic changes in the organ. As Ayurveda says there are three causes of functional disorders—wrong use, non-use and over use. Though Ayurveda has described the causes in a nutshell but could not explain them in detail. As regards the eye, Dr. W.H. Bates of America gives a fine description about the wrong use, non-use and over use of the eyes which often cause errors of refraction and many other defects of the eye. The methods that cure such functional defects can be studied from Mind and Vision. I herewith illustrate the subject with interesting case reports.

### Wrong Use

1. READING: A lady aged 18 years complained of frequent headache in reading. The eyes felt great strain even in reading one page. At times headache became severe and to relieve this headache she took 'Anacin' tablets. On examination it was found that she had normal vision both for distance and near. Her health was fine. But while she was reading I noted two wrong habits in her. She held the book at about 20 inches from her eyes and she did not blink even once in reading the whole page.

I said, "Are you an old lady?"

She was annoyed, "Why do you say so, doctor?"

"Because you hold the book at a distance where usually old people keep it."

She replied, "But my grandfather frequently warns me to keep the book at a long distance so that sight may not deteriorate."

"Yes, your grandfather is an old man, he cannot focus at a near distance. The normal distance for young people is between ten to twelve inches."

When the lady held the book at about 12 inches she found the print distinct and clearer.

To correct the other mistake I taught her how to blink gently. In blinking the upper lid comes a little down and is again raised. Blinking should not be mistaken into winking in which the upper lid touches the lower lid. Winking is bad for the eyes, while blinking is very helpful and relaxing. One may blink about five or ten times a minute. When this patient adopted the right habit of blinking while keeping the book at about twelve inches, she could read for hours without any discomfort. The principle is that one should hold the book at a distance where the print is seen best. The distance is immaterial. Myopic patients would like to keep the book nearer. To make her eyes still stronger I advised her to read fine print in dim light as well for a few minutes daily as an exercise to the eyes.

WRITING: Some years ago a Rani had consulted me at Mussoorie where I had gone for summer resort. She showed me several pairs of spectacles and eye remedies. Her complaint was severe headache which usually appeared while writing or seeing cinema show, and to relieve this headache she had to rest for hours in her bed. She was observing that memory was being affected.

Her eyesight was normal and the eyes were quite healthy. General health was also good. I could not detect any cause of her headache. Then I asked her to write dictation. After writing a few lines she began to feel little discomfort and immediately the mistake was caught. She was writing forward and at the same time trying to read the back letters already written, and this is a wrong method of using the eyes. The right way is to move the sight with the movement of the pen and avoid reading of back letters and words. To check the wrong habit I gave her a piece of blotting paper with which she covered the back letters while writing and thus she could write page after page without any discomfort.

CINEMA: Now the next problem was how to cure headache which troubles her while seeing the cinema. Usually when a patient complains of headache or discomfort in some particular work, I tell the patient to repeat the work in my presence. She showed me how she looked at the picture and that was the expression of strain. I told her to adopt the right way. When she kept her chin a little raised and the upper lids downwards so as to keep the eyes half open in the posture of rest, she could blink gently while seeing the picture. After that she immensely enjoyed the cinema and told her friends about the wonderful method of seeing the cinema.

SEWING: Many women suffer from headache and eye strain in needle work. This trouble is not usually due to weak eyesight but due to bad visual habit. Recently a girl complained of headache and eye strain in sewing. She was wearing glasses and following the doctor's instructions rigidly, but there was no relief. She had adopted a wrong way of sewing, that is, she kept her sight fixed on the cloth and neither she moved her sight with the movement of the needle nor she blinked.

But when she adopted the right method of sewing, she felt great relief. The right method is to move the sight with the movement of the needle; when the needle comes up, the sight comes up; and when the needle comes to the cloth, the sight shifts to the cloth. She then continued sewing without her glasses and felt no discomfort. In fact, fine stitching is an aid to eyesight, when it is done in the right way.

## Non-Use

When one does not use the eye consciously or unconsciously, functional disorder takes place. It is a common experience that the eyes become sensitive to bright light after remaining in a dark room for some time. The eyes are not used in the dark room.

A boy was almost blind with his right eye though the eye in its structure was quite normal. On examination it was found that he was neglecting to use the right eye unconsciously. Such a condition is called amblyopia, and many cases are found suffering from amblyopia. Such cases are usually supposed incurable but by relaxing the mind and eye education the patient can greatly improve his vision. This boy had very good memory and could recall the actual image in his imagination while palming. The result was that he could improve his vision to normal in a very short time.

## Over Use

Reading for many hours at a stretch causes excessive accommodation and when the students look at distant objects after reading for long hours they are unable to focus correctly at distant objects. Under such a condition when there is a strain to see the distant object they develop short sight. A boy had normal eyesight at the age of ten years but later on developed myopia, as he had the habit of reading for long hours, late in the night, and while seeing distant objects he had developed the habit of staring as he could not adjust his focus at a distance quickly. This is why many voracious readers, particularly students, develop myopia. Some escape because some how they are able to relax the eyes and can adjust the focus correctly both at the near and at the distance. Even if the distant objects are not clear, they do not make an effort to see, they shift the focus to nearer objects.

## Effect of Solar Eclipse Upon the Eye

When one looks at the sun with open eyes, it is usually the heat of the sun which is harmful to the eyes. This is why the Acharyas recommended to observe the solar eclipse or face the sun while bathing in a tank or a river. The blood circulating became cool and heat was eliminated. Similarly it is recommended to see the image of the sun in water or use smoked glass. Any harmful effect after seeing the solar eclipse can be relieved soon by putting cold cotton pads or cold mud packs on the eyes or by relaxation of the mind.

A college student stared at the solar eclipse for about fifteen minutes with both eyes open. Just after seeing the eclipse everything seemed to be blurred, covered with smoke. Next day something like a whirling flower composed of white and dark specks appeared all the time before the eyes even when they were closed. Whirling was very fast for the first three days. On the fifth day the patient felt a black speck bigger than the sun before his eyes all the time. While seeing sign-boards, sticks, parallel bars or other straight things, he felt them distorted. The lines of the book print seemed to be curved and the letters dim. The black speck varied in size according to the distance he fixed his sight. He consulted many doctors and their opinion was, "A part of the retina was burnt, and the defect would remain permanent. Use dark glasses." After examining the eyes of this patient, I explained to him that my opinion differed. The resulting blind area (scotoma) and other symptoms were not due to any organic change but were the result of a strain of the mind and eyes while seeing the solar eclipse. A return to normal was quite possible, and the prompt relief of the symptoms mentioned would follow the relief of eye strain. When the mind is perfectly relaxed, nothing can harm the eyes and sight. By relaxation of the mind some persons can look at the sun for sufficient time without any discomfort or loss of vision.

My conversation impressed the patient and he was confident now about his cure. He had a good memory and it seemed to me easy to help him because good memory is a great aid to eyesight if it can be rightly applied. When he closed the eyes and covered them with the palms, avoiding any pressure on the eyeballs, I asked him if he could imagine that he was writing his name with pen and black ink on a sheet of white paper. He said he could do it quite easily. I directed him to spell his whole name and then imagine each letter, and to place an imaginary dot at the end of his name. I asked him next to forget about his name and remember the dot. The patient was able to remember the dot and remarked that the dot appeared to move in various directions with a short, slow, easy swing. Memory of dot may be difficult for many patients and other relaxation methods may be tried in such cases. After ten minutes when the patient opened his eyes he felt a cooling sensation in his eyes and relief of his discomforts. He frequently closed the eyes and covered them with the palms for ten or fifteen minutes each time, and usually remembered a black dot but sometimes he liked to recall the memory of other things as the colour of his black shoes and white trousers and his familiar game badminton.

While practising on the Snellen test card the patient glanced at the white centres of the letters instead of fixing the sight on the blackness of the letters. At times he closed the eyes for a minute or longer, remembering white snow, white paint, a white cloud in the sky. This enabled him to observe that the white centres of the letters appeared whiter than the margin of the card, and as the white centres appeared whiter, the blackness also increased, and subsequently the letter became perfectly distinct. His reading sight was soon improved when he moved his sight on the white spaces in between the lines of print without making any effort to look at the letters. Blinking was a great help. At times wet cold pads were put on the eyes and the eyes were bandaged. Sun treatment was avoided and medicines were applied locally.

Within a few days the sight became normal, and distortion of straight things disappeared, but the black speck faded gradually and it took one month when the speck disappeared completely.

(2) Another patient, a Sannyasi, having normal vision stared at the mid-day sun just to attain some abnormal power. After a few minutes when he took the sight away from the sun he began to see the sun on everything which he saw. When he closed the eyes, the sun was visible in his imagination. This became a great discomfort to him because the true form and colour of the object was not visible due to the appearance of the sun on the object. Reading and writing became almost impossible. It was declared by the doctors that the condition

of his eyes could not be improved as the retina of his eyes was damaged.

The Sannyasi was a man of determination and he dared to challenge the opinion of doctors. In the night when the moon was shining brightly he looked at the moon for at least an hour with the idea that the cooling rays of the moon would neutralize the effect of the hot rays of the sun. While looking at the moon he mentally imagined the moon. The Sannyasi made himself all right within three days. To confirm that his discovery about the treatment was genuine he again made his eyes worse by looking at the sun. Again he repeated his experiment and looked at the moon in the same way and made his eyes all right.

## EYE EDUCATION

### Blinking and Winking

LOOK at the eyes of a tiny baby who has a natural impulse to blink, look at the eyes of a cow or a dog or an elephant, they all blink. The upper lid comes a little down and is again raised, it does not touch the lower lid in the action of blinking. Blinking is a continuous habit of good eyes. By blinking the eyes work under rest, the habit of staring is checked. While reading one should blink at each line, while seeing some distant object shift the sight from part to part and blink.

What is winking? In winking the upper lid touches the lower lid with a jerk. Look at those who have bad eyes. There is a tendency to stare. Blinking is absent or it is done at long intervals or the person winks instead of blinking. Winking is bad for the eyes. It is a sort of disease. Winking is conspicuous while blinking is not conspicuous.

Blinking helps to relieve the strain and to improve eyesight. Look at the Snellen test card placed at ten feet, read it without blinking and note down the result. Now read it while blinking gently at each letter and note down the result. You will observe that your vision is recorded better when you read the eye chart with blinking. Another thing, gaze at a letter of the chart or a figure of a calendar at ten feet, don't blink, observe that the letter begins to fade. Now look at it with gentle blinking and you can see it continuously without losing its clearness. So blinking is very essential for the preservation of good eyesight.

*How to develop the habit of blinking?*

1. Take two pencils one in each hand. Keep one at six inches and the other at arm's length. Look at the tip of each pencil alternately. You will observe a short movement of the lids. This will teach you how much the lids should move in right blinking.

2. Place a mirror before you. Look at the right eye and blink. Look at the left eye and blink. It will keep you aware of right or wrong blinking.

3. Walk and blink at each step observing that the ground appears to move backwards. This will give you the habit of frequent blinking.

4. Take some small print and shift the sight on white lines in between the lines of print and blink at each white line, in good light and candle light. This will improve your eyesight and will act as a strong preventive to all sorts of eye ailments. You will observe that the print becomes clearer while shifting the sight on white lines.

A boy somehow had developed the habit of staring, he did

not blink at all while reading or seeing distant objects. Often he made mistakes in reading as the letters and words either became double or disappeared. He was semiblind. It is simply by blinking and frequent palming that normal eyesight was restored.

Another case, the patient of high myopia, having lost much of his vision due to progressive myopia attended the School for Perfect Eyesight. His very look of eyes indicated that he keeps the lids steady and stares at objects without a blink. Often he suffered from pain and headache. How much soothing it was and how much helpful it was when he looked at things with gentle blinking and read the blackboard with short movements of the lids.

All defective eyesight cases should learn blinking if they want to improve their eyesight. Even if glasses are necessary, blinking should be done to prevent further deterioration. Persons suffering from glaucoma have a very strong bad habit of staring. It is usually very difficult for them to adopt the right habit of blinking. However, if they can be taught to blink frequently in the right way, their trouble of glaucoma will be cured or at least reduced much.

Greatest things are always simplest. Blinking is very simple, and it will be found that a great deal more reading can be done with blinking than without it, and also the eyes will not be tired.

## READ THE NATURAL WAY

A lady patient while on educational tour to U.S.A. was experiencing some difficulty in reading and writing. Her eyes quickly tired and became prominent as if protruding from the bony socket, a horrible appearance quite disfiguring to the face.

At times while reading the words appeared double and often she made mistakes in transcription. She had to give up the work of stitching as sewing was very uncomfortable. There was a constant feeling of dryness and heaviness in the eyes. Often her lady friends laughed at her inability to match the colours while selecting some cloth. She had developed the habit of staring while reading or seeing different objects. At times the pain and headache became severe and she had to rest long hours. The glare of the sun was very unpleasant and when she moved in an unknown place she got knocks as her field of vision was contracted.

When Khorshed put these visual difficulties before the eye specialists at U.S.A. they found her eyes quite normal. They could not think that these visual defects could be due to mental strain and wrong use of the eyes. They put her to different tests and the conclusion was that her eye troubles were due to hyperthyroidism. When she returned to India, Bombay doctors supported the diagnosis and treatment of U.S.A. doctors and gave thyroid orally but there was no relief to her eye troubles.

Finally Khorshed left herself at the mercy of the divine grace. One morning she was on a visit to Sri Aurobindo Ashram and had an opportunity to visit the School for Perfect Eyesight. She is an intelligent and charming personality hence it was necessary to tell her frankly that it was a mistake of over specialists to collaborate the visual defects with the thyroid disorder. Both were quite separate troubles. Hence the treatment of thyroid failed to give any relief. I explained to her that the eye being a sense organ was closely associated with the mind in its functioning. The strain of the mind would immediately affect the eyesight, while the relaxation of the mind would benefit the eyes. To demonstrate this fact she was asked to stand before a window with vertical bars in it. When she moved the body, head and eyes to the right while raising the left heal she observed that the bars of the window appeared to be moving to the left and vice versa. As soon as she practised this swing in the right way she felt greatly relaxed but when she practised the swing in the wrong way, she felt a great strain in the eyes and head.

Another great difficulty was that she did not blink. She did not know how necessary it was to blink gently to keep the eyes at rest all the time. It was difficult at first to adopt the right habit of blinking but by the application of different relaxation exercises and bandaging she could train her eye lids to blink in a normal way.

When the sight is perfect the subject is able to observe that all objects regarded appear to be moving. A letter seen at the near or at the distance appears to move slightly in various directions. The pavement comes towards the person in walking, and the side houses appear to move in the opposite direction. In reading, the page appears to move in a direction opposite to the movement of the eye. If one tries to imagine things stationary, the vision is lowered and the discomforts and pain may be produced. By observing the movement of lines while shifting the sight on white lines in between the lines of print, Khorshed felt a great relief and could read and write for a long period without any discomfort. In sewing she shifted the sight with the movement of the needle. To overcome the glare of the sun she faced the sun for a few minutes daily.

Whenever Khorshed looked intently at a letter or an object she felt fatigue and discomfort and the object blurred or became double. There was a feeling of tension in the eyes and head. To break this habit of staring she was taught the following:

1. Shift consciously from one part to another of all objects regarded, and imagine that these objects appeared to move in a direction contrary to the movement of the eye.

2. Look at the blackness of the letter for a second and close the eyes for half a minute while recalling the memory of black. When she practised successfully, the memory of blackness increased. Then she did palming for sufficient time till she felt her eyes greatly relaxed.

3. Looking towards the candle flame while counting one hundred respirations soothed her nerves greatly. While reading fine print she moved her body forward and backward.

## GLASSES AND EYE EDUCATION

IT is a fact that glasses enable people to see well at a distance or near, but this is also true that glasses become an added torture to increase pain and suffering and loss of sight in many cases. The fast deterioration in eye sight and the development of some serious complications are not prevented by the use of glasses, injections and pills. Therefore, the number of blind people amongst the educated class is increasing fast inspite of all possible medical aid. All such cases of threatened blindness can be greatly benefited by eye education and mental relaxation exercises. If the children and adults are taught about the proper use of the eyes, most of the defects of eye sight will fade away in due course of time.

The orthodox belief that for errors of refraction there is not only no cure, practically no preventive also, is based on fallacies and any rational mind will think such a claim as dogmatic, an imperfection in the science. When the sight begins to deteriorate, there must be some cause for it. And the cause is always an effort to see or strain. Strain to see at a distance causes myopia, while strain to see at the near point causes hypermetropia. Glasses neutralize the effect of such errors of refraction but don't relieve the cause of trouble. So in many cases the cause continues increasing by the use of glasses and the sight goes on deteriorating. Unless the prescription of glasses is supplemented by eye education, deterioration in eyesight and blindness will continue to increase.

It is time that some doctors should carefully study the subject of eye education as discovered by Dr. W.H.BATES, M.D. the Pioneer Ophthalmologist of New York and repeat his experiments if necessary. If this can be done in the spirit of a true scientist, then the Indian doctors will have a distinguished place in the comity of nations. They will be regarded as saviour of the human race. The Ophthalmic Science will advance fast and the notion of the incurability of eye defects will fade away and we will be able to discover some definite means to prevent and cure blindness which is often due to low or high tension glaucoma, Retinitis Pigmentosa or some other retinal degeneration.

All along it has been my experience that mental relaxation is the key of success in life and in education, and treatment. Under the present civilized conditions man's mind is under a severe strain, hence preservation of good eyesight is almost impossible without eye education and mental relaxation. Dr. Bates has made many remarkable discoveries for the prevention and cure of defective eyesight. To promote his thought and spread the scientific knowledge the SCHOOL FOR PERFECT EYESIGHT has been opened under the auspices of Sri Aurobindo Ashram, Pondicherry. The School provides a four years course in Ophthalmic Science which is based on the synthesis of various systems of medicine, with Dr. Bates system of eye education as the main scientific path-pointer.

Then our future doctors will bring quick recovery by their simple and harmless methods. Their very presence will vibrate a sense of ease, comfort and relief.

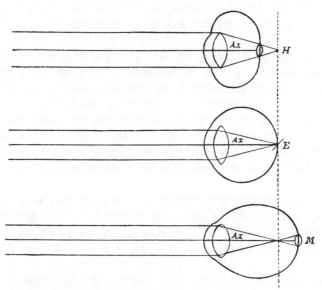

H, Hypermetropia ;    E, Normal eye;

M, Myopia. Note that in hypermetropia and myopia the rays, instead of coming to a focus, form a round spot upon the retina.

# CHAPTER VII

## ANCIENT WISDOM IN OPHTHALMOLOGY

THE history of two thousand years ago tells us about the merits of Indian Medicine. Sushrutta, the seer, thinker, physician and surgeon was the first Indian Ophthalmologist of that time who wrote about Ophthalmology. In his book 'Sushrutta Samhita', the author has described Ophthalmology in a concise and simple way. Of course, nothing is mentioned there about glasses and methods of relaxation. The fundamental principles of treatment are convincing and helpful. Some truths for the prevention and cure of eye troubles are also found in other Indian texts like Gita, Mahabharata, Upanishads, Charak-Samhita etc. Although the scientific basis is forgotten today, the old truths survive in the form of religious practices.

The discoveries of modern science in the sphere of medicine and surgery, the rectification of defective vision by glasses etc. are amazing. But it has to be admitted that our modern methods, however efficient as palliatives, generally fail to prevent and cure errors of refraction or floating specks or eye strain and headache, which sometimes lead to serious complications. A careful study of the subject reveals that unless the modern knowledge is supplemented by other methods having the stamp of scientific truth, cases of defective eyesight and eye troubles would greatly increase. In the ancient medical literature and allied books one can find simple practices and things to prevent and cure errors of refraction, to strengthen the eyes and treat effectively other serious diseases of the eye.

According to Indian Medicine there are three fundamental principles of treatment—Elimination, Stimulation, Relaxation—about which a reference is already made in the preceding chapters. A patient usually needs the application of all the three principles in varying degree, but in some patients elimination and in others stimulation or relaxation may be the primary need, though the trouble may be the same. For example, a patient feels great eye strain and headache. If the strain is due to constipation then purgative or enema will prove useful, but if the strain is due to lack of vitality then tonics will relieve the trouble. Or if the trouble is due to staring or lack of sleep, then relaxation and rest will cure the patient. The art of applying these principles can be acquired through experience and a certain 'intuition'.

## Therapeutic Agents

1. USE OF HONEY: Honey is a viscid, semi-transparent liquid yellowish brown colour, of aromatic odour and sweet acrid taste, prepared by the honey-bee.

Indian medicine lays great stress on the use of honey for application in eye troubles. Honey is supposed to be valuable remedy in non-inflammatory conditions to relieve disorders and strain of the eye. It stimulates the mucous membrane and acts as a vaso-dilator and lymphagogue. Its power to stimulate vascular and lymphatic circulation renders it of great value in the treatment of large number of ocular diseases. Honey is used preferably in its pure form and is applied in the eyes as an ointment and its action is increased if the person faces the sun (early or last in the day) for about five minutes with eyes closed just after its application. It is often combined with other remedies as sodium chloride, onion juice, ginger juice, copper sulphate etc. in the treatment of defective vision, eye strain, floating specks, night blindness, retinitis, early optic atrophy, incipient cataract, early glaucoma and opacity cornea. Its application in the eye causes a little burning sensation followed by slight redness and watering. These symptoms disappear in a few minutes.

2. OCULAR SUN THREAPY: According to Indian tradition, as found both in scientific treatise and religious texts the sun is regarded as 'God of the eyes' (Chakshu Devata). By facing the sun regularly in a proper manner, the eyes gradually become bright, shining and attractive. The vitality of the eyes is greatly increased and microbes cannot usually harm eyes. Inflammatory conditions and other discomforts of the eye are greatly relieved.

The Ophthalmologist of today is afraid of giving sun rays to eye patients and various methods are adopted to protect the organ of vision. The evidence on which this almost universal fear of sunlight has been based is, I believe, of flimsy character. In the rather extensive literature on the subject one is confronted with such a lack of scientific truth that in 1910, Dr. J. H. Parsons of the Royal Ophthalmic Hospital of London addressing a meeting of the Ophthalmological section of the American Medical Association, felt justified in saying that Ophthalmologists, if they were honest with themselves 'must confess to a lamentable ignorance of the conditions which render bright light deliterious to eyes' (JOURNAL OF AMERICAN MEDICAL ASSOCIATION, December 10, 1910, p. 2028.)

In the School for Perfect Eyesight almost every patient is advised to face the sun with the eyelids closed and sway the body gently from side to side like a pendulum to relieve monotony for about five minutes when the sun is not hot. This simple process has been found by clinical experience to be highly beneficial. After sun treatment the eyes are washed with saline or cold water.

Sun treatment with open eyes is also advised in selected cases, especially of opacity cornea. The patient covers the head with a napkin, keeps the feet in a basin full of cold water and looks at the morning or evening sun with frequent gentle blinking while moving the body from side to side like a pendulum. After open eye sun treatment washing the eyes and face with cold water is very refreshing.

3. CONCENTRATION: Concentration and meditation are traditional Indian methods as the daily routine of each individual. This is designated in the ancient vocabulary as "Sandhya", which means nothing more and nothing less than the practice of concentration i.e. centering the thought on one object of devotion or contemplation both morning and evening. In many Vedic passages the Rishis who were seers or men of vision are said to 'see with their mind' (*Manasa Pashyanti*). Modern Ophthalmology frankly recognises the value of the mind as operative agent of vision, although its external instrument is a normal healthy eye.

In the Indian scriptures it has been repeatedly mentioned that eyes are sensory organs and perform their function normally without effort; what we see is the interpretation of the retinal images by the mind. When the mind is under strain as in fear, worries etc. and the eyes make an effort to see, the vision is affected. In this age of the increasing prestige of psychosomatic medicine it should not be difficult to accept the ancient wisdom about the influence of the mind or spirit on the sight. Seeing is a complex process depending on five factors as Charak mentions in his Samhita—object of seeing, organ of sight, sense function, interpretation of mind and attention of inner mind. To see perfectly the eye should have full contact with the object to see. Then the external mind should be at rest so as to give correct interpretation. Then the inner mind should pay attention to see the object. The eye without the mind will mechanically photograph the image but will not interpret it. The mind without the eye can imagine the images previously seen, but will not tell you what you are seeing now. Correct seeing must be a perfectly coordinated action between mind and eye.

To relieve the strain of the mind and eyes, concentration with eyes closed has been recommended. Every one might have observed that when the eyes are tired simply closing the eyes rests them and clears the vision. Greater relief is obtained when the eyes are closed and covered with the palms of the hands, avoiding any pressure on the eyeballs, for a few minutes. Dr. Bates calls this practice 'palming'. When the eyes are closed and covered one may develop concentration by recalling the memory of pleasant, familiar and interesting objects without effort and if the imagination is according to the reality the eyes and mind are greatly relaxed, the strain is relieved and the vision improves. When palming is successful one feels all dark before the eyes when they are closed and covered, and this darkness may be compared to black printer's ink. During warm weather hands may be washed with cold water so as to make them wet while palming.

4. TRATAK ON OM-CHART: Tratak is the ancient Sanskrit word for Central Fixation and has been practised in India on Om to maintain perfect sight or to improve the defective vision. In the Om Chart inside the circle there is the word 'OM' which is written in the traditional manner symbolising the supreme vital power in creation. The exercises practised with it develop the sensitiveness of central spot of the retina (macula lutea), acuity of vision and increase blood circulation. The macula lutea is the most sensitive part of the retina and the eye

sees best through this area. The result is that the letter or part of a letter of Snellen test card on which eye fixes itself appears most distinct. This quality of the eye is called Central fixation. But when the sight is imperfect, for whatever cause the sensitiveness of the macula and central fixation are always affected. When the eye possesses central fixation it not only possesses perfect sight, but it is perfectly at rest and can be used indefinitely without fatigue. Loss of central fixation means strain, and when it is habitual leads to all sorts of abnormal conditions and is, in fact, at the bottom of most eye troubles. By improving the central fixation the vision soon begins to improve but the limits of improvement depend upon the degree of central fixation. The following practices on Om chart and Snellen eye test card help in improving central fixation and the benefits already observed are, in short so great that the subject merits further investigation.

*Practice No.* i. Fix your eye at the commencing point of the central figure ॐ and note that the part you look at appears clearest. Then shift the sight slowly on the rest of the character; note all the time that the portion of it seen appears darkest. Repeat the practice three times and observe that the whole character appears of darker shade. The practice may be done at i foot to io feet.

*Practice No.* ii. There are angular lines all round; shift the sight on the angular lines and note that the line regarded is seen darkest. As the sight moves on the lines the head also moves. The head and eyes should shift together and gentle blinking ought to be maintained. This may be done at i foot to 5 feet.

*Practice No.* iii. There is a circular line around. ॐ Shift the sight along with the head and eyes on the circle with eyes open and then with eyes closed in your imagination. When

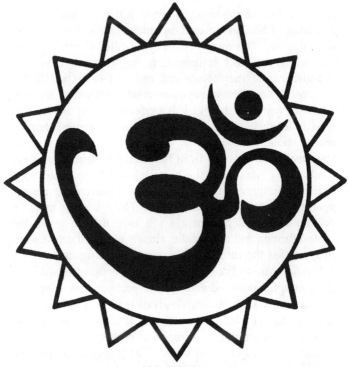

OM CHART

done properly, proves very helpful especially in cases in whom the eyeballs become more or less stationary as in glaucoma and retinal diseases.

*Practice No.* IV. Take one Snellen test card. Shift the sight from bottom to top and top to bottom of a letter. Suppose the letter of the Snellen test card is C. Now regard the bottom part of the letter C and note that the top part of C is less distinct, then shift the sight to the top part of C and note that the bottom is less distinct. Repeat three times. Then close the eyes for a few seconds and repeat the practice on the smaller letters.

5. FINE PRINT AS AN AID TO EYE SIGHT: It may not be generally known that the finest writing was practised in India in a number of manuscripts of religious texts, like the Gita, the Bhagwata and the Mahabharata. Such texts were intended for daily recitation. They served the same purpose as is at present served by the photographic type reduction.

Ancient India was also famous for its fine embroidery, stitching, painting and sculpture and it is said that most people who performed very fine knitting work maintained good eyesight throughout their life. This practice indicates that fine work may be an aid to eyesight. I have found fine print reading as an aid to eyesight. Persons who often complain of headache and strain, or whose reading sight is gradually failing, or whose number of reading glasses is gradually increasing, are greatly benefited by reading of fine print or diamond type. Those who cannot read it without glasses, may read it with glasses. Even shifting the sight on the white lines in between the lines of print is an aid to eyesight. Reading of fine print or photopgraphic type reduction daily when it can be done without discomfort, has invariably proved to be beneficial.

### Seven Truths of Normal Sight

1. Normal Sight can always be demonstrated in the normal eye, but only under favorable conditions.
2. Central Fixation: The letter or part of the letter regarded is always seen best.
3. Shifting: The point regarded changes rapidly and continuously.
4. Swinging: When the shifting is slow, the letters appear to move from side to side, or in other directions with a pendulum-like motion.
5. Memory is perfect. The color and background of the letters or other objects seen, are remembered perfectly, instantaneously and continuously.
6. Imagination is good One may even see the white part of letters whiter than it really is, while the black is not altered by distance, illumination, size, or form, of the letters.
7. Rest or relaxation of the eye and mind is perfect and can always be demonstrated.

When one of these seven fundamentals is perfect, all are perfect.

### CHAPTER XIII

#### MEMORY AS AN AID TO VISION

WHEN the mind is able to remember perfectly any phenomenon of the senses, it is always perfectly relaxed. The sight is normal, if the eyes are open; and when they are closed and covered so as to exclude all the light, one sees a perfectly black field —that is nothing at all. If you can remember the ticking of a watch, or an odor or a taste perfectly, your mind is perfectly at rest, and you will see a perfect black when your eyes are closed and covered. If your memory of a sensation of touch could be equal to the reality, you would see nothing but black when the light was excluded from your eyes. If you were to remember a bar of music perfectly when your eyes were closed and covered, you would see nothing but black. But in the case of any of these phenomena it is not easy to test the correctness of the memory, and the same is true of colors other than black. All other colors, including white, are altered by the amount of light to which they are exposed, and are seldurs seen as perfectly as it is possible for the normal eye to see them. But when the sight is normal, black is just as black in a dim light as in a bright one. It is also just as black at the distance as at the near-point, while a small area is just as black as a large one, and, in fact, appears blacker. Black is, moreover, more readily

### Specimen of Fine Print & Photographic Type reduction

6. TARPANA: Tarpana is a kind of eyewash which Sushrutta employed in the treatment of various eye diseases to relieve the strain and pain, to soften the tissues, to produce vitality and to increase the sensitiveness of the retina. The patient laid on his back in a room not exposed to the rays of the sun and gust of wind, and a circular ring of a particular kind of paste was made on the eyelids. Then the mixture of old clarified butter and luke warm water was poured in the eyes and retained there for a few minutes. Afterwards the paste of barley flour was applied on the eyes for about an hour. In my institute I have modified this process of Tarpana according to the modern conditions and is given to special cases.

*Things required*: Sterilized eye cups, clarified butter to which camphor 10 grains to an ounce has been mixed by heating, warm distilled water, cotton pads, paste of coarse barely flour, bandage.

*Time of Tarpana*: Afternoon when it is neither very hot nor very cold.

*Process*: At first the eyes are given hot fomentation or vapour bath. Then take luke warm water in the eye cup and add to it about 1 dram of camphorated clarified butter and mix with a rod. The patient will wash his eye in it for about two minutes. After the eye wash a pad having barley paste over it is put on the eye and light bandage is applied which is kept on the eye for one or two hours. The process is repeated for three to five days usually. The petient is warned not to expose the eyes to the source of light or bright light, fire, sky, looking-glass or any other luminous object, and blast of wind.

*Symptoms of defective Tarpana*: Cloudiness in vision, heaviness, lacrimation, itching, photophobia, excessive glossiness.

*Symptoms of satisfactory Tarpana*: Good sleep, cessation of secretion, clearness in vision, agreeable sensation, lightness in the eyes.

*Treatment of defective Tarpana*: Remove constipation, give vapour to the eyes and apply Anjana prepared from camphor smoke.

*Cases fit for Tarpana*: Falling of eye lashes, cloudiness of vision, errors of refraction specially high myopia, retinal diseases, hardness of eyelids.

# Chapter VIII

# DIETETICS

Foods promote growth of the body and repair and its waste, yield material energy for muscular and brain work, yield heat, regulate body processes and make reproduction possible. According to the modern idea, fuel and energy foods are carbohydrates, fats and proteins; foods that build the cells are proteins and salts, while regulators of body processes are minerals and vitamins. On this basis many concentrated and highly valuable foods have been discovered and there is so much good literature on the subject, yet the modern doctor usually feels something missing when he tries to prescribe adequate diet to a patient. Ayurveda fills up this gap to a great extent by prescribing diet according to tastes. There are six tastes—sweet, sour, alkaline (salty), pungent, bitter and astringent. For health all the tastes are necessary but their use is to be adjusted in diseases.

SWEET TASTE: All cereals, milk, butter, oils, sweets, meat, egg, bonemarrow, banana, dry fruits, fruits of sweet taste as apple, grape, sugar cane, potato etc. According to modern knowledge proteins, fats and carbohydrates are included in sweet taste.

Sweet taste articles enrich nutrient fluid, blood, flesh, bonemarrow, bone formation, vitality and semen. It relieves thirst, and heat; gives complexion to skin, hair; gives stength to sense organs; and it is liked by bees and ants.

Much use of sweet taste articles causes fatness, softness of muscles, lethargy, hypersomnia, weakness of gastric fire, cough, cold, constipation, vomiting, mucus, sweet taste in the mouth etc.

SOUR TASTE: All citrate fruits as lemon, organge, prunes, peaches, pomegranate, tamarind, mango etc.

Sour taste gives relish to dishes, stimulates digestive fire, helps in building up body cells, invigorates heart, produces salivation, conducts the food downwards and moistens the food.

Much use of sour taste articles increases thirst and heat, causes watering in the eyes, vitiates blood and causes œdema in emaciated and debiliated patients. On account of its acidity it leads to suppuration of inflammations and wounds. It causes all round burning sensation in throat, chest and heart.

ALKALINE TASTE: This includes salts as sodium chloride, soda bicarb, black salt, ammonium chloride, leafy green vegetables as they contain more salt.

Alkaline taste articles are diffusive, digestive, laxative, curative of stiffness, help in removing obstruction and accumulation of toxic matter, liquify mucus secretions and give relish to food.

Much use of salt causes heat and thirst, impairs the function of sense organs, forms premature wrinkles and grey hair.

PUNGENT TASTE: This includes pepper, chillies, ginger, cinnamon, cloves, long pepper, asafœtida, onion etc.

Pungent taste purifies mouth, increases gastric fire, causes watering from the eyes, sharpens sense organs, curative of intestinal sluggishness, odoema and obesity, eliminative of excretory matter, dilates passages, removes mucus.

Much use of pungent articles causes emaciation, giddiness, burning sensation and heat, and distroys manhood.

BITTER TASTE: This includes karela (bitter gourd), neem, chirata etc.

Bitter taste is appetising, purifies blood, curative of burning, itching, thirst and dermatosis. Hence very useful in inflammations and suppuration, skin diseases and diabetes and leprosy etc.

Much use dries nutrient fluid, blood etc. and affects the nerves.

ASTRINGENT TASTE: This taste includes pomegranate, rasot, alum, jambul, Amla (Eblic myrobolan), Harr (Myrobolan), Bahera (Myrobolan beliric), mango seed etc.

It is sedative, soothing, efficacious in inflammatory conditions, peristalsis, diarrhœa, stomatitis etc.

Much use dries mouth, efflicts throat, impedes speech, constricts blood vessels, intestine and ureters etc.

## Prescription of Diet According to Season

DURING WINTER: In winter appetite is increased on account of increased gastric fire due to flow of blood to internal organs, hence take sugar, fats, oils, wheat, rice, milk, oil massage, warm water, sun bath.

Avoid cold drinks, restricted diet, pungent, bitter and astringent articles when one is quite healthy.

DURING SPRING: After winter sun rays become hot, and heat liquifies the toxic matter in the body. This is why people suffer from cold, fever etc. Hence eliminative procedure is useful. Avoid free use of sugar, fats and oils. Add pungent, bitter, astringent and alkaline articles. Physical exercise is very helpful.

DURING SUMMER: Increased heat of the sun dries up the body fluid, hence foods and drinks that are sweet, cool, liquid and unctuous are good. Ghee, milk, curd, sugar, old rice and old wheat are preferred.

DURING RAINY SEASON: Digestive power is weakened hence

moderate diet is preferred. Honey is very useful. Avoid watery and demulcent drinks, day sleep, sun bath.

DURING AUTUMN: After rains heat is increased. Ghee with bitter articles is very good. Avoid exposure to sun.

## Light and Heavy Articles

LIGHT ARTICLES: Light articles stimulate gastric fire and satisfy hunger and thirst.

Rice, green gram, salt, barley, milk, honey, fruits, vegetables, meat juice, soup, butter-milk, sago, ghee in small quantity, cooked rice soaked in cold water for about four hours etc.

HEAVY ARTICLES: Heavy articles are roborant and increase blood and flesh.

Wheat, black gram, butter or ghee, cream, cheese, meat, egg, fish, pastry, sweetmeats, puddings, dry fruits, dates, nuts etc.

## Dietetic Rules

1. Hot food invokes digestive fire.
2. Ghee excites inactive gastric fire.
3. Eating measured quantity according to one's digestion does not disturb digestion.
4. Eat after the digestion of previous meal.
5. Masticate well and avoid talking and laughing but eat with due concentration.
6. Eat in a clean place.
7. Do not eat in an enemy's house.
8. After meal chew cloves, cardamom, betel-nut etc. for salivation and fragrance.
9. After meal rest or walk gently; sitting posture is not good; do not move in fast vehicles if they cause great jerk.

10. When there is fatigue after physical exertion, always take rest and then take meal.

## Effect of Measured and Good Diet

1. No discomfort in stomach and heart.
2. Subsidence of hunger and thirst.
3. Sense of ease in standing, walking, lying, breathing etc.

## Evils of Inadequate Diet

1. Deficient diet causes impairment of strength and vitality.
2. Eating solid in excess in addition to drinks irritates the stomach and humors, and causes disorders.
3. Untimely eating of heavy, cold and dry things causes disorders.
4. Eating unclean and incompatible articles are harmful.
5. Eating when mind is affected causes indigestion.

## Harmful Diet

1. Food not taken according to gastric fire.
2. Combination of ghee and honey in equal parts.
3. Drinking hot water after taking honey or eating warmed honey.
4. Use of cold and hot things at a time as ice cream and tea.
5. Eating cold things after taking fat preparations as cold drink after fried articles.
6. Food under cooked, over cooked or burnt.
7. Sour things with milk or food unpleasant to taste.
8. Juice of unripe, over ripe or putrified substances.
9. Half curdled curd.

To relieve any harmful effect give purgatives and emetics for quick relief.

NOTE: When digestion is quite good and gastric fire is strong, any diet can be taken without any harmful effects, but when the digestive fire is weak or the person is of sensitive nature, harmful effects of inadequate diet usually manifest. At first the symptoms of disorder manifest in the digestive system as indigestion, constipation, gastritis, diarrhoea, etc. Afterwards other organs are affected due to sluggish liver and inadequacy of kidneys.

## Qualities of Articles

GROUP A CEREALS

1. RICE—Sweet, cooling, diuretic, unctuous, forms condensed and scanty stools.

2. BARLEY—Sweet, cooling, dry, increases faeces, eliminates mucus.

3. WHEAT—Sweet, cooling, unctuous, heavy, vitaliser, roborant.

4. HORSE GRAM—Sweet, dry, hot, eliminative.

5. GREEN GRAM—Sweet, dry, cooling, light.

6. BLACK GRAM—Sweet, heavy, aphrodisiac.

NOTE: Pulses cause flatulence and are dry,
hence must be taken with pungent, salt and ghee.

GROUP B VEGETABLES

1. GREEN LEAFY VEGETABLES—Eliminative, laxative and digestive.

2. CUCUMBER—Powerful diuretic.

3. KARELA (Bitter gourd)—Stimulates liver, purifies blood.

4. POTATO—Hot and dry, hence should be taken with ghee.

5. ONION—Appetising, relieves flatulence.

6. GARLIC—Hot and aphrodisiac, curative of worms, dermatitis and leprosy.

7. BOTTLE GOURD AND LUFFA (Loki and Toroi)—Cooling.

8. LADY'S FINGER (Bhindi)—Demulcent, eliminative and nutritious.

9. TOMATO—Blood purifier.

## GROUP C—FRUITS

1. APPLE—Sweet and cooling, very good in diarrhoea.

2. ORANGE—Acid and cooling.

3. FIG—Nourishing and laxative.

4. MANGO—Hot, stimulates liver.

5. POMEGRANATE—Astringent, curative of phypersecretion of mucus, inflammations and hyperaemia.

6. DATES—Heavy, hot, roborant, beneficial in wasting and trauma.

7. GRAPE—Sweet and cooling, quickly relieves thirst and burning in fever.

## GROUP D

MEAT JUICE—Most nourishing, increases semen and complexion.

MILK—Vitaliser; very good in fatigue after fasting, travelling, lecturing etc. Best after meal. Goat's milk helpful in consumption. Buffalo's milk induces sleep and lethargy. Cow's milk preferable.

BUTTER-MILK—Light, useful in assimilation disorders and

suppression of urine.

FRESH BUTTER—Digestive, astringent. Useful in trauma, anorexia etc.

CURD—Appetiser, digestive stimulant, recommended in diarrhoea and dysentery, irregular faeces and anorexia etc. Curd is prohibited in cold and coryza. Immature curd delays digestion.

TIL OIL—Relieves discomforts of flatulence and pain. Its gargles increase sense of taste and the strength of teeth.

## Diet in Diseases

INFLAMMATORY CONDITIONS as acute ophthalmia, iritis, scleritis, conjunctivitis, glaucoma etc.

In inflammatory conditions the principle is to give dry and eliminative diet with less sugar avoiding hot and acid things. Such a diet helps to reduce the tension and inflammation.

Take whole wheat bread, barley, horse gram, unpolished rice, green gram.

Take all vegetables with less potato.

Fruits in less quantity. Roasted horse gram about 2 to 4 ounces daily and water as little as possible.

Avoid milk, ghee and their preparations and citrate articles.

PURULENT DISEASES as dacryocystitis, hypopeon, ulcer cornea, purulent conjunctivitis, panophthalmitis etc.

Here the principle is to give bitters with reduced sugar.

Wheat, barley, rice, horse gram, green gram are good.

All vegetables especially bitter gourd, and all fruits.

Butter with pungent articles as ginger and black pepper.

Salad, curd, sweet oil, olive oil.

Avoid sweetmeats and milk.

DEBILITY AND NIGHT BLINDNESS

Such patients need diet as a tonic hence rich diet is preferred according to the gastric fire.

All cereals with butter or ghee.

Fresh butter mixed with little black pepper and sugar every morning. Or almonds 5 to 20, soaked in water and skin removed, to be taken with dry grapes or some such preparations.

Rice with ghee, milk and honey.

Milk heated with red hot rings of gold and then mixed with ghee, honey and sugar.

Fish fried and egg.

Enema with sweet oil, meat juice, milk, sugar and honey.

Cod liver oil, Triphala ghrita, Vitamin A preparations.

ERRORS OF REFRACTION

Generally these cases are normal in digestion and health and a change of diet is not necessary. However, nourishing diet as milk, butter, almonds are very good.

CHRONIC DISEASES OF RETINA as retinitis, retinopathy etc.

Usually these dieases happen in old people in whom digestion and assimilation become weak. Constipation is a general disorder and diabetes is present in most cases. Here the principle of diet is eliminative, light with pungent and bitter articles.

Wheat and barley, unpolished rice, more green leafy vegetables, milk, salad, fruits.

Drinking of a few drops of lemon in water several times a day.

Karela juice every morning. Pickles and pepper allowed.

TRIPHALA GHIRTA—1 teaspoon Triphala, ½ teaspoon butter, ½ teaspoon Sugar (See Triphala on page 96.)

Mix and take with a cup of warm milk at bed time daily or twice a week.

ASSIMILATION DISORDERS

Symptoms—Large quantity of stools, bitter and acid eructations, thirst, loss of strength, heaviness and loss of appetite.

Treatment—Purgation, fast, drinking water with lemon drops or soda bicarb or fruit juice.

After elimination light food with digestive stimulants, buttermilk, fruits.

Persons who pass dry stools with difficulty should take ghee with salt in the midst of meal.

When digestion is weak eating of garlic with oil, or ginger with salt, or asafœtida with ghee before meals.

INCREASED APPETITE AND GASTRIC FIRE

Milk pudding, ghee preparations, sweetmeats, dry fruits, wheat preparations.

THIRST

If thirst is due to heat, give water with sugar and lemon, syrup, milk, Thandai etc.

Thirst due to rich food is quenched with jaggery and water.

Thirst due to high fever is quenched with dry prunes.

In anaemia, abdominal diseases, coryza, catarrhal conditions, urinary diseases, weak gastric fire, diarrhoea, drinking water in the least quantity is helpful. In such cases coriander water with honey or sugar is very good.

## STOMACH—INTESTINE WASH

Stomach-intestine wash is a Yogic process to keep the body fit, free from most of the physical and mental ailments especially in old age.

1. Drink 3 or 4 glasses of lukewarm water (about 2 litres) to which common salt has been added to make the water saline. Then stand with 60 degree angle, put the fingers in the throat and try to vomit. If vomiting does not take place then leave it. If vomiting has taken place then drink one or two glasses of warm saline more.

2. After that do not rest in the bed. Walk and try the following exercises with ease so that saline may pass down quickly and easily.

a. Stand with the feet about one foot apart, raise the hands up, clasp them together and move the hands from side to side. The muscles of the abdomen will be felt stretched.

b. Stand about one foot apart, raise the arms at right angles to the body and move the arms in semi-circular direction, about ten times.

c. Lie down on the abdomen, palms on the ground, then raise the head and chest and look upwards towards the ceiling—repeat about ten times.

d. Stand about one foot apart with a bent body and move the muscles of the abdomen forward and backward. After each exercise walk gently and repeat again till you feel to pass motion. After about half an hour there will be solid clear motion.

3. After the motion again drink one or two glasses of warm saline water and again repeat the above exercises. This time there will be semi-solid motion after about half an hour.

4. After the motion again drink one or two glasses of warm

saline and repeat the exercises. This time there will be yellow liquid motion with sufficient mucous in it.

5. Again drink one or two glasses of warm saline and repeat the exercises. This time there will be watery motion with a yellowish tinge in it.

6. No more to drink. There will be a feeling of dryness in the system. If you like you may massage the body with oil and have a good warm bath.

7. After about two hours of bath when you feel quite hungry take well cooked *KHICHRI* a preparation of 2 parts green gram pulse and one part of rice. Add to it at least two ounces of ghee or butter, mix well. Eat slowly. Do not take curd or milk till next day. Do not drink cold water and do not sleep till the diet has been taken.

The feeling will be of warmth in the body and upsurge of energy vibrating in the whole body.

8. This process may be repeated once a month when you are on a holiday. If you start at 6 a.m. then about six hours will be spent in the whole process.

# CHAPTER IX

# CLASSIFICATION OF ORGANIC DISEASES OF THE EYE

To classify the organic diseases of the eye Sushruta has used the terms Vataja, Pittaja, Kaphaja and Tridosha type of diseases.

Vataja means Painful or paralytic diseases.

Pittaja means Inflammatory diseases.

Kaphaja means Non-inflammatory diseases.

Tridosha means Purulent or degenerative diseases or diseases having unusual symptoms.

1. *Vataja Type of Diseases*: All painful or paralytic diseases are classified under this heading. The nerves go under a strain and there is lack of relaxation. The following are some of the Vataja type of diseases:

| | | |
|---|---|---|
| Painful glaucoma | or | *Hata-adhimantha* |
| Neuralgic pain | or | *Anyato-vat* |
| Blepharospasm | or | *Nimesha* |
| Paralysis lid or Ptosis | or | *Vat-hat-vartama* |

2. *Pittaja Type of Diseases*: Diseases in which there is irritation, burning, redness, watering are classified under this heading.

| | | |
|---|---|---|
| Acute conjunctivitis | or | *Pittaja Abhishanda* |
| Redness due to acid fruits | or | *Amladhyushita* |
| Scleritis and iritis | or | *Adhimantha* |
| Congestion, pannus | or | *Sira-harsha* |
| Keratitis | or | *Sukra-roga* |
| Stye | or | *Anjanahari* |

3. *Kaphaja Type of Diseases*: Non-inflammatory dieseases or having mucoid discharge are in this list.

| | | |
|---|---|---|
| Silent glaucoma | or | *Kaphaja Adhimantha* |
| Simple conjunctivitis | or | *Kaphaja Abhyshanda* |
| Mucoid cyst | or | *Balasa-granthi* |
| Pterygium | or | *Shuklaarma* |
| Big cyst | or | *Lagna* |

4. *Tridosha Type of Diseases*: Diseases in which there is purulent discharge or the degenerative changes are taking place or the form and function completely disorganised, are classified under this heading.

| | | |
|---|---|---|
| Chronic dacryocystitis | or | *Puyalasa* |
| Panophthalmitis | or | *Akshipakatya* |
| Boil | or | *Utsangini* |
| Purulent conjunctivitis | or | *Kardma Vartma* |
| Staphyloma | or | *Ajaka* |
| Night blindness and colour blindness | or | *Nakulandhya* |

Sushruta has also classified eye diseases according to the part affected. A large number of diseases have been added by the modern Ophthalmology but I give here a list which Sushruta has written.

## Diseases of Eye Lids

| | |
|---|---|
| Blepharitis | *Kumbhika* |
| Odoema of the lid | *Vartma-Bandha* |
| Inflammatory swelling | *Klishto Vartma* |
| Chalasion | *Utsangini* |
| Stye | *Anjanahari* |
| Ptosis | *Vat-hat-vartma* |
| Trichiasis, entropion | *Pakshma-kopa* |

| Blepharospasm | *Nimesha* |
| Herpes | *Pothaki* |
| Trachoma | *Arsho-vartma* |
| Follicular conjunctivitis | *Shushkrasas* |
| Cyst | *Lagna* |
| Chronic dacryocystitis | *Puyalasa* |
| Excessive itching with glare and lacrymation in a child | *Kukunaka* |

## Diseases of Sclera and Conjunctiva

| Pterygium | *Shuklaarma* |
| Fleshy growth | *Lohitaarma* |
| Pinguicula | *Snavarma* |
| Sub-conjunctival haemorrhage | *Suktika* |
| Scleritis | *Arjuna* |
| Extensive redness, pannus | *Sirajala* |
| Phylectenular conjunctivitis | *Shirapidaka* |

## Diseases of Cornea

| Ulcer cornea | *Savrana Shukra* |
| Opacity cornea | *Avrana Shukra* |
| Panophthalmitis | *Akshipakataya* |
| Staphyloma | *Ajaka* |

## Diseases of the Whole Eyeball

| Ophthalmia | *Abhishandya* |
| Chronic ophthalmia with pain and headache | *Adhimantha* |
| Silent glaucoma, optic atrophy, blindness due to pain and | |

| | |
|---|---|
| headache | *Hataadhimantha* |
| Vision cloudy, glare, lids dry and hard | *Shushka akshipaka* |
| Swelling of eye due to acid fruits or acid reaction | *Amladhyashita Drishti* |
| Deep inflammation as ch. iritis, cyclitis, uveitis | *Shirotapata* |
| Blindness with redness in the eye and pannus as in glaucoma | *Shiraharsha* |

## Diseases of Pupil

| | |
|---|---|
| Cataract | *Katcha* |
| Cataract, glaucoma | *Linga-nasa* |
| Clouded pupil | |
| Night blindness | *Shleshma-vidagdha drishti* |
| Smoky vision | *Dhum drishti* |
| Colour blindness or appearance of various colours before the eye | *Nakulandhya* |
| Contracted and deformed pupil as in synechia | *Gambhirika* |

# LINE OF TREATMENT IN ORGANIC DISEASES

**Elimination:** 1. Remove constipation by purgative, enema or by adding green leafy vegetable and fruits in diet.

2. Drop errhine in the nose as Sharbindoo oil especially in inflammatory conditions and chronic conditions

3. Educate the eye how to relieve wrong habits of seeing by gentle blinking, etc.

**Stimulation:** 1. Prescribe suitable diet and tonics when needed.

2. Sun treatment and vapour.

3. Tarpana.

**Relaxation:** 1. Frequent palming and reading finer print with gentle blinking.

2. Swinging and central fixation exercises.

3. Bandage.

Operations and glasses when necessary.

Apply medicines as eye ointments, eye wash and drops, Anjana or surma.

## A Few Important Hints

1. When there is acute inflammation of the eye with intolerable pain as in acute ophthalmia and actute glaucoma, fomentation should not be given on the eye but around the eye; also relieve the congestion and tension by giving strong purgative as Brooklax and drop an errhine in the nose to bring out discharge.

2. When there is excessive pain in the eye or head without inflammation, usually the principle is to prescribe fatty substances in diet as well as for local application. Use castor oil as purgative and Sharbindoo oil as errhine. Educate the patient to relax by palming and swinging.

3. When discharge is excessive with inflammation, give purgative and some errhine to drop in the nose. Diet should be light avoiding sour and hot articles. If there is burning sensation, never apply irritants to the eye, soothing applications are more helpful. Avoid bandage especially if the discharge is thick.

4. When there is strain in reading, give fine print to read with or without glasses preferably in dim light.

5. In an organic disease having any visual defect, the function is also disturbed. In most cases the trouble starts as functional disorder or loss of central fixation, and later on it becomes an organic trouble. So the eye should be educated to adopt the right function by central fixation exercises along with necessary treatment for the organic trouble. By doing so the organic defect may continue but there will be improvement in vision and general condition of the eye.

6. Avoid operation when the eye is under acute inflammation or acute pain. Relieve the crisis by other means.

7. Irritating medicines causing much watering are to be applied towards the evening or at bed time.

8. Sun treatment with closesd eyes is generally very helpful in eye troubles.

9. Avoid atropine drops unless very necessary.

10. Ointments containing fatty substance are usually to be applied in the evening or at bed time otherwise greasy layer on the cornea causes glare and discomfort.

## Treatment of Headache

1. In most cases headache is due to wrong use of the eyes as in reading, writing, seeing cinema, sewing, driving, parties, marketing, travelling, etc. The patient will tell that headache comes under such and such condition. Right education of the eyes will cure the headache. Study *Mind and Vision*.

2. Many cases of headache are due to mental strain and eye strain. Frequent palming and reading fine print will relieve headache. Head massage is also good.

3. Some patients complain of headache when they put on glasses. Probably the number is not correct or the eyes resent.

4. Headache coming in the morning after sleep and dis-

appearing after a short while, is due to mental strain during sleep. Palming and long swing before and after sleep very helpful. Touch swing gives wonderful results in some cases.

5. In some cases headache appears from sunrise to sunset or after sunset in the night. Patient likes dashing the head against a wall. It may be half sided, hemicrania. Errhines are very helpful.

6. If headache after supression of cold, sneezing powder, Sharbindoo oil in the nose or saline douche are very good.

7. When headache due to heat as after moving in the sun, cold bath and cold drink are very good. If after some exhaustion, give warm milk and palm. If due to exposure to cold, take hot tea or Banaksha tea and rest or a pill of aspro. Head massage.

8. Headache due to constipation, fever or some other physical trouble needs medical treatment. Head massage.

9. When headache after illness and there is feeling of dryness in head, nose and ears, give nourishing diet as halwa, harira, rice with sugar and ghee, almonds etc. Drop oil in the nose and ears. Nasal douche with milk may be given. Head massage.

10. When headache due to descent of higher force, rest and silence, palm.

11. Severe headache first felt in one of the temples followed by red swelling and burning pain, the whole head affected, affecting voice; it is called in Ayurveda SANKHAKA. If not treated properly may cause death or severe damage to head and eyes, usually optic atrophy.

Treatment—Cooling plasters on head, nasal drops, snuff, drinking ghee through nose, sprinkling of cold water or goat's milk on head, apply ghee washed 100 times on head. If constipated, strong enema.

Probably yellowish poison is formed and accumulated in the brain substance; first headache appears in the temple and then spreads.

Following changes usually happen in headache:

1. Blood gets hot, capillaries distended, congestion.

2. Brain cells get irritated and strained.

3. Subtle energy in the body unable to neutralize the effect of the heat.

**Zone Therapy:** Press the thumb or some metal instrument as the handle of a large knife, firmly as you can against the roof of the mouth under the seat of headache for 3 to 5 minutes.

# Chapter X

## SYNTHETIC EXPOSITION

THERE are four well-known systems of medicine—Ayurveda or Indian Medicine, Allopathy or Modern Medicine, Homeopathy and Nature Cure. The follower of any one system is usually dogmatic. The conservative mind tries to measure things by a standard it has set up in its intelligence and views things from a single standpoint. It is not able to harmonise different ideas and view the facts from different standpoints. But Nature has her subtle and disguised methods in her dealings with men by which she leads them to change.

In fact each system is a part of the whole, discovered by man as the necessity arose. Hence a synthesis is possible. Each system has its limitations and a harmonious combination of good points of each system based on a central principle common to all will be called a synthetic system of treatment. Such a system I have formulated for eye troubles but this can be worked out for the rest of the body troubles on the same lines.

**Ayurveda:** Ayurveda gives a simple and scientific conception of man and philosophy of medicine. Its simple prescriptions of herbs etc. prove very efficacious and harmless in many disorders of the body especially in humoral disorders and when elimination of the toxic matter in the form of motions, urine, vomiting, perspiration, and nasal discharge, is the primary need in the treatment. Principles of dieting are very good. Prevention and cure of infectious and parasitic diseases are lacking. Methods of investigation are inadequate. There is no treatment for many functional disorders as errors of refraction, squint etc. Nothing has been mentioned about glasses which are a necessity to many. Surgery is in its infancy. Necessarily this system is to be considerably supplemented.

**Allopathy:** This system is a progressive one and has discovered novel and highly scientific methods of investigation. The modern scientific instruments, X-rays, the knowledge of bacteriology and bio-chemistry have proved very helpful and enabled a student to do research work. The discovery of glasses and the technique of their application have enabled many to see clearly from distance and near. The operative technique has given an additional value to this system. The treatment of infectious and parasitic diseases, discovery of Penicillin, cortisone, sulphanomide drugs, Chloromycetine, vaccine and serum etc., have greatly attracted the public attention. Yet Allopathic science is an infant science. Although the modern doctor has made many remarkable discoveries he has failed to prevent and cure a simple error of refraction or cure a simple case of cold. Many diseases of the inside of the eyeball are supposed to be due to syphilis and focal infection and antisyphilitic or antitoxic treatment is adopted but the results are very poor, even there is no prevention. The poor results are due to the failure in determining the true causes of such eye diseases. Similarly, theory of glaucoma, floating specks and accommodation etc., are very confusing. In the treatment the eye is usually isolated from the mind and the body, and attention is paid mostly to local and physical means which often do not yeild good results.

**Homeopathy:** Homeopathy believes that there is a healing energy or life-force which cures sickness. This energy is already present in the body and many diseases and many patients are cured without any treatment. It is through this life-force that the body survives in sickness, imparts the faculty of feeling and controls the functions of life. In sickness this life force is primarily deranged and its effects are made known by abnormal feelings and functions which appear in the body in the shape of symptoms of a disease. If this life force can be strengthened by the artificial drug force of the same nature (Similinum), the body throws off the abnormal sensations and symptoms and thus the cure is effected.

Its sweet medicines in very minute doses are usually inno-cent and efficacious though to many its subtle way of treatment is not appealing. When the primary need in the treatment is to stimulate the life-force, its medicines prove very helpful but their usefulness depends on the person who prescribes and also on the effectivity of the medicine. If the physician has a primary good intention of healing a patient and is able to transmit his thought power through the medicine, the action of the medicine will be very effective. Right selection of the medicine is also needed and to become a successful Homeopath intuition is much more helpful than the intellectual knowledge. There are a great number of medicines and the treatment is followed according to the symptoms in the individual. This requires a great study and experience and probably rare indi-viduals can be called successful Homeopaths.

**Nature Cure:** In this system there is more stress on enema, cold and hot baths, steam bath, sun bath, massage, physical exercises, yogic asanas, breathing exercises, regulation of diet, control over desires and passions, formation of correct habits, concentration, eye exercises through rest and relaxation. Attention is greatly paid to relieve the strain of the eye and mind to improve the vision. Proper application of these methods gives quick relief and remarkable results but some cases do need medicines or glasses or operation and this aspect we have to supplement from Allopathy, Ayurveda and Homeopathy.

**Synthetic System:** A synthetic system should consider all the systems of treatment and collect all the good points from each. From Ayurveda we can adopt its simple philosophy, simple methods of elimination and treatment, various good prescriptions, principle of dieting. Allopathy provides the scientific knowledge of investigation, prescription of glasses, technique of operations, treatment of parasitic and infectious diseases, some very useful medicines and injections. Homeopathy gives the idea of stimulating the life-force in sickness. Nature cure enlarges the field by physical and relaxation exercises.

Such a synthetic system of treatment is being practised in Dr. Agarwal's Eye Institute, at Delhi and Madras and in the School for Perfect Eye sight. The value of its efficacy and practical working has now become widely known. Most of the cases, so called incurable, are benefited considerably by simple and harmless methods of treatment. A report of such cases appeared now and then in medical journals.

I give here a few cases as an illustration.

**Case No. 1:** A man of forty four was suffering from eye troubles for over thirty years and had consulted Allopaths, Homeopaths and Ayurvedic physicians. His main troubles were pain in the eyeballs, headache, occasional redness and dimness in near work. Whenever there was an attack of redness he had to stop his work and remain in the room for days together.

Doctors had treated him by itrritant medicines and prescribed glasses for constant use. Homeopaths had given some internal medicines. Ayurvedic physicians had prescribed some purgatives, tonic and Surma. The patient had temporary relief, a sort of suppression of the symptoms but he was conscious of gradual deterioration in eyesight. The present condition was pterygium in the right eye, slight redness, old age sight, floating specks before the eyes, pain and headache especially in near work. After a thorough examination with retinoscope and ophthalmoscope the patient was treated on the following lines based on synthetic system. In the treatment three principles—elimination, stimulation and relaxation—were adopted.

| | |
|---|---|
| Elimination: | Prescribed Triphala preparations as a purgative (Ayurveda) |
| | Operation of pterygium (Allopathy) |
| Stimulation: | Triphala ghrita as a tonic (Ayurveda) |
| | Saline eye wash (Allopathy) |
| | Anjana or surma for application in eye (Ayurveda) |
| | Sun treatment and central fixation exercise (Nature cure) |
| Relaxation: | Relaxation exercises for the eye and mind (Nature cure) |

Prescription of glasses for near work (Allopathy)

The results were remarkable. His distant vision became normal and required lower power of glasses for reading. Complaints of pain, headache, redness and floating specks disappeared. The expression of the eyes became normal.

Case No. 2: An indoor patient had an attack of malarial fever and there was great restlessness. To relieve this restlessness a Homeopathic medicine 'Aconite 30' was given and just within a few minutes all the restlessness turned into good sleep. Then in the morning an enema was given to clear the bowels, and a few small doses of quinine mixture stopped the malarial fever.

Case No. 3: My son suffered from typhoid fever and I knew that this fever will take at least 21 days provided there was no complication. To shorten the time of suffering and quick recovery I gave the boy enemas, cold hip baths, saline to drink for vomiting during the first four days according to Nature cure. On the sixth day when it was decided by laboratory test and in consultation of other doctors that the case was of typhoid fever, Chloromycetine capsules were started along with Vitamins and liquid diet according to Allopathy. After twenty four hours the temperature came down and on the tenth day the boy was quite all right.To keep the head cool ghee washed 100 times accordng to Ayurveda was kept on the head and it was surprising how quickly this ghee (clarified butter) was soaked.

## Medicines

Prescription of medicines has two aspects—one is temporary and the other is permanent. For example, Charak based the whole philosophy of Ayurveda on Tridosha and discovered many herbs for treatment. The later physicians found that the metal therapy or Rasa Chikitsa was more powerfully effective than herbs, so they began to prescribe metal therapy but its prescription was based on Tridosha. So the temporary aspect is herbal treatment and the modes of its application, while Tridosha on which the prescription of drugs is based is an eternal aspect of medicine. The temporary aspect goes on changing according to the times and today many Ayurvedic physicians have begun to use injections, and other drugs discovered by the Western mind but the principles on which they prescribe such things are the same.

In medicine there are a multitude of remedies but a small number are of proven value. A large number are of slight or questionable value. Certain drugs and formulae find favour with some physicians while others they never receive a trial. One great danger in medicine is the falling into a therapeutic rut. The preservation of an open mind, and willingness to give a trial to the untried, is a valuable asset. We should warn against the therapeutic nihilist on the one hand, and the extreme enthusiast on the other. The remedies should not be strong and violent but such as are beneficial without disturbing the organ or the body, and the dose should be as small as possible. Most old prescriptions containing numerous constituents can be simplified and still maintain the same effect. In most cases simple prescriptions and simple instructions regarding relaxation are more than sufficient if the physician understands the principles and the art of healing properly. We have simplified many Ayurvedic prescriptions or modified them according to the present conditions.

## Ancient Methods of Investigation of Drugs

1. Rasa: It means description of actions of a drug through its taste. Many things when tasted reveal their taste and according to the taste the actions and therapeutic uses have been described and this simple process has greatly simplified the treatment of humoral disorders and the prescription of dieting.

2. Guna: It means the description of actions of a drug through the sense of touch and sight. A thing may be heavy or light, fatty or non-fatty, dry or moist, soft or hard, hot or cold, coarse or smooth in texture, solid or liquid in shape etc. Just as the Acharyas saw and felt they described the qualities of a drug and on this basis they described the possible actions of it. For example, heavy things like pulses, wheat relieve the pain of appetite and make the body strong. Fatty things as clarified butter, almond oil etc. relieve the dryness of skin and give strength to the nerves. Any green vegetable helps in clearing the motions.

3. VEERYA: Observation of action of a drug when it reaches the stomach by chewing or swallowing is termed as Veerya. By this method it was determined whether a thing was an irritant or non-irritant, stimulant or depressant, created heaviness or lightness in the body, increased gastric secretion or not, produced cooling sensation or hot sensation, whether it acted as an emetic or not. On this basis they prescribed ghee, salts, asafœtida etc. to increase the gastric secretion, digitalis as an stimulant, madanphal as an emetic.

4. VIPAKA: Actions of some drugs were determined when they were digested and absorbed, and this method is termed as Vipak. It was determined whether a drug increased the blood and acted as a tonic or not, whether it helped in the elimination of toxic matter and whether it had any sedative action etc. Thus it was observed that meat, bone-marrow, honey etc. acted as a tonic. Aloin, Triphala, senna and guava helped in the elimination. Opium and dhatoora had sedative action.

5. PRABHAVA: When a drug acted differently and the reason of its action could not be explained, then this process was termed as Prabhava.

MODERN METHODS: Science has much advanced due to highly developed intellect and has discovered some very remarkable drugs. The scientists have used microscope and other laboratory methods to discover the actions of a drug or they have produced quite a different combination by chemical actions. For example, dhatoora dilates the pupil and opium contracts the pupil. The modern methods have shown that dhatoora contains atropine alkaloid which dilates the pupil, while opium contains eserine which contracts the pupil. These ingredients have been separated from dhatoora and opium by modern methods and how useful they are as eye remedies. Today we see Penicillin, a derivative from a plant, widely used in many Tridosha cases. In this way modern scientists have discovered many wonderful drugs and their methods of application. Thus a failing heart can be quickly stimulated by an injection of digitalis and strychnine, a serious attack of malaria can be challenged by quinine, diptheria can be cured within twentyfour hours by anti-diptheric serum. Gonorrhoea can be cleared within a few days by Penicillin. And so on.

# CHAPTER XI

## MEDICAL PRESCRIPTIONS

### Eye Wash

THE eye cup is a popular means for washing the eye. Fill the cup with water and add to it a few drops of the eye wash solution by the dropper. Then put it against the eye gently. Its lower margin touches the lower eyelid while the upper margin remains free. Keep the eyes downwards and gently blink while washing the eye. Wash each eye for about two minutes or more. The following eye-wash solutions may be used:

| | | | | |
|---|---|---|---|---|
| 1. Sodium chloride | ... | ... | ... | ... grain X |
| Soda bicarb | ... | ... | ... | ... grain X |
| Distilled water | ... | ... | ... | ... ounce I |

10 to 20 drops of it are added to an eye cup full of water.

| | | | |
|---|---|---|---|
| 2. Soda biborate (Borax) | ... | ... | ... grain VI |
| Soda bicarb | ... | ... | ... grain VI |
| Sodium chloride | ... | ... | ... grain VI |
| Witch Hazel (Hazeline) | ... | ... | minim XCVI |
| Distilled water | ... | ... | ... ounce IV |

Take water, preferably lukewarm, in an eye cup and add to it 20 to 30 drops of this lotion. Wash the eye as directed above. This is a soothing eye wash and is very useful in simple conjunctivitis.

3. Sodium chloride ... ... ... ... grain LX
   Cold boiled milk ... ... ... ... ounce VIII

Useful in conjunctivitis, trachoma and redness in the eyes.

### TRIPHALA

4. Amla—Eblic Myrobolan
   Harr—Myrobolan
   Bahera—Myrobolan Beliric

Prepare 'Triphla' by taking equal parts of Amla, Harr and Bahera. Wash them with water and then dry. Prepare coarse powder. Take one tea-spoonful of this powder and add to it two ounces of water. Let it remain for the whole night in a small earthen or glass pot with a cover on it. Filter the lotion in the morning and use it for eyewash. Very useful in redness of the eye.

5. Honey ... ... ... ... ... dram II
   Sodium chloride ... ... ... ... dram I
   Milk ... ... ... ... ... ounce IV

This is a tonic eye wash for dull and weak eyes.

### Eye-drops

1. William's Modified Drops
   Cocaine nitrate ... ... ... ... grain ½
   Boric acid ... ... ... ... grain XII
   Sodium borate ... ... ... ... grain X
   Camphor water ... ... ... ... dram II
   Distilled water ... ... ... ... ounce I

This is an agreeable and soothing eye-drop to use after silver nitrate, zinc or other irritating drops have been instilled.

2. Collyrium Flavum

| | | | | |
|---|---|---|---|---|
| Phenol | ... | ... | ... | grain I |
| Fluid extract of hydrastis | ... | ... | | minim II |
| Witch hazel water | ... | | ... | mininm XXX |
| Boric acid | ... | ... | ... | grain X |
| Distilled water | ... | ... | ... | ounce I |

These drops have a momentary sting, which is replaced by a cool, pleasant sensation.

3. Zinc drops

| | | | | |
|---|---|---|---|---|
| Zinc sulphate | ... | ... | ... | ... grain I |
| Distilled water | ... | ... | ... | ... ounce I |

This is very useful in conjunctivitis, especially when little secretion is present.

4. Camphor Drops

| | | | | |
|---|---|---|---|---|
| Acid tannic | ... | ... | ... | grain $^1/_4$ |
| Zinc sulph. | ... | ... | ... | grain $^1/_2$ |
| Aqua Camphor | ... | ... | ... | dram II |
| Distilled water | ... | ... | ... | ... dram IV |

Useful in simple conjunctivitis.

5. Silver Nitrate Drops

| | | | | |
|---|---|---|---|---|
| Silver nitrate | ... | ... | ... | grain II |
| Distilled water | ... | ... | ... | ounce I |

Useful in conjunctivitis and trachoma.

6. Argyrol Drops
   Argyrol       ...        ...        ...     ... grain X
   Distilled water    ...      ...        ...     ... ounce I

Useful in conjunctivitis and trachoma.

7. Atropine Drops
   Atropine sulphate    ...        ...     ... grain II
   Distilled water    ...      ...        ...     ... ounce I

These drops dilate the pupil and are chiefly indicated in
irits for dilating the pupil.

8. Eserine Drops
   Eserine salicylate    ...        ...        ...     grain I
   Distilled water ...        ...        ...     ... ounce I

Eserine drops diminish the size of the pupil and are used
chiefly in glaucoma.

9. Pilocarpine Drops
   Pilocarpine nitrate    ...        ...     ... grain II
   Distilled water  ...        ...        ...     ounce I

These drops also contract the pupil and are used in glaucoma.

10. Cocaine Drops
    Cocaine Hydrochloride    ...      ...    grain IV
    Distilled water    ......      ...      ...    dram II

Cocaine Drops are commonly employed for producing local
anaesthesia during operations upon the eye.

11. Antiseptic Drops

| | | | | |
|---|---|---|---|---|
| Mercurochrome | ... | ... | ... | grain IV |
| Distilled water | ... | ... | ... | ounce I |

Useful in acute conjunctivitis and ulcer cornea.

12. Adrenaline Drops

Liquid adrenaline is a valuable astringent and haemostatic. It is used in operations. It proves very useful in subjective conjunctivitis.

| | | | | |
|---|---|---|---|---|
| 13. Sodium chloride | ... | ... | ... | dram I |
| Dry ginger powder | ... | ... | ... | dram $^1/_2$ |
| Milk | ... | ... | ... | dram VII |

These Drops are very useful in smoky vision, retinitis, night blindness, retinopathy, choroiditis and early optic atrophy.

14. Penicilin Drops

Take a phial of crystaline Penicilin. Add to it 10 c.c. of distilled water. Take 1 c.c. out of it and add 4 c.c. distilled water to this 1 c.c.
Very useful in conjunctivitis or in any infectious condition of the eye.
In acute conjunctivitis drop the lotion frequently.

15. Cortisone Eye Drops or ointment

These are ready made eye drops. Useful in iritis, iridocycilitis, keratitis.

16. Sodium Sulphacetamide Drops

  Sodium Sulphacetamide ...  ...  ... grain 30
  Distilled water ...  ...  ... ... dram II

Very useful in trachoma. To be dropped 3 or 4 times a day.

HONEY APPLICATIONS

Medicines prepared in honey prove very useful. They are applied to the eye by a rod. Their application just before the sun treatment proves very efficacious. *Resolvent* 200, *Resolvent* 500 and *Opacitox Occulose* are the patent medicines of Dr. Agarwal's Eye Institute made with honey.

1. Sodium chloride ...  ...  ... grain XXX
  Honey ...  ...  ...  ... ... ounce I

Useful in defective eyesight, floating specks, after cataract operation.

2. Dionin ...  ...  ... ... ... grain X
  Honey ...  ...  ...  ... ... ounce I

Useful in defective eyesight, opacity cornea, early cataract.

3. Sodium chloride ...  ...  ... grain XXX
  Sulphate of iron ... ... ...  ... grain XXX
  Honey ...  ...  ...  ... ounce I

Useful in old pannus.

4. Onion juice ... ... ... ... dram I
   Ginger juice ... ... ... ... dram I
   Honey ... ... ... ... ... ounce I

Useful in night blindness and diseases of the retina and choroid.

5. Chandrodaya powder (Ayurvedic preparation) dram I
   Honey ... ... ... ... ounce I

Useful in cataract, opacity cornea, trachoma.

6. Sea foam ... ... ... ... dram I
   Conch shell ... ... ... ... dram I
   Sodium chloride ... ... ... dram I
   Honey ... ... ... ... ... ounce IV

Useful in opacity cornea and early cataract.

POWDERS OR SURMAS OR ANJANA
   1. Menthol ... ... ... ... grain VIII
      Black antimony ... ... ... ... grain XX
      Calomel ... ... ... ... dram IV

Useful in defective eyesight, spring catarrh, scleritis, conjunctivitis and trachoma.

2. Black antimony ... ... ... ... ... dram I
   Potassium nitrate ... ... ... ... dram I
   Camphor ... ... ... ... ... grain VI

Useful in defective eyesight.

3. Sodium chloride ... ... ... dram IV
   Turmeric (Haldi) ... ... ... dram I

Useful in night blindness and diseases of the retina.

4. Kajal or black powder ... ... ... dram I
   Menthol ... ... ... ... ... grain III
   Camphor ... ... ... ... grain III

Useful in conjunctivitis and for beauty.

5. Sea foam ... ... ... ... ... dram I
   Sodium chloride ... ... ... dram I
   Conch shell ... ... ... ... dram I
   White pepper ... ... ... ... dram I

Very useful in itching of eyelids, chronic conjunctivitis with mucoid discharge, especially in children, in opacity cornea.

6. Copper sulphate ... ... ... grain XV
   Asafœtida ... ... ... ... dram II
   Dry ginger powder ... ... ... dram II
   Sodium chloride ...... ... ... ounce III
   Black antimony ... ... ... ounce I

Very useful in Kaphaja conjunctivitis with mucoid discharge.

7. Mamira of China ... ... ... dram II
   Copaiba ... ... ... ... dram II
   Calomel ... ... ... ... ... ounce II

Very useful in weak eyesight, dullness of the eyes.

# OINTMENTS

## 1. Aristol Ointment

| | |
|---|---|
| Aristol ... ... ... ... ... | grain I |
| Olive oil ... ... ... ... ... | minim XV |
| Lanoline ... ... ... | ounce I |

Of service after injuries, burns and operations.

## 2. Atropine Ointment

| | |
|---|---|
| Atropine sulphate ... ... ... | grain I |
| White vaseline ... ... ... | dram II |

Of service for dilating the pupil and in iritis.

## 3. Atropine and Dionin Ointment

| | |
|---|---|
| Atropine sulphate ... ... ... | grain I |
| Dionin ... ... ... ... | grain II |
| White vaseline ... ... ... ... | dram II |

Of great service in iritis and iridocyclitis.

## 4. Boric Ointment

| | |
|---|---|
| Boric acid ... ... ... ... | grain IV |
| White vaseline ... ... ... ... | dram II |

Applied in conjunctivitis at bed time.

## 5. Copper Citrate Ointment

| | |
|---|---|
| Copper citrate ... ... ... | grain I |
| White vaseline ... ... ... ... | ounce I |

Useful in chronic conjunctivitis and trachoma.

6. Menthol Ointment

| | | | | |
|---|---|---|---|---|
| Menthol | ... | ... | ... | grain V |
| White vaseline | ... | ... | ... | ounce I |

Useful in conjunctivitis and trachoma.

7. Sulphonamide Ointment

| | | | | |
|---|---|---|---|---|
| Sulphonamide powder | ... | ... | grain XXX |
| White vaseline | ... | ... | ... | ... | ounce I |

Useful in conjunctivitis, trachoma, ulcer cornea etc.

8. Terramycine ointment and Aureomycin ointment are available in ready made tubes and are very useful in trachoma and conjunctivitis.

9.

| | | | | |
|---|---|---|---|---|
| Alum | ... | ... | ... | ... | dram VI |
| Opium | ... | ... | ... | ... | dram I |
| Butter (cow) | ... | ... | ... | ounce IV |

Put the butter in iron pan, and let the butter melt. Then add powdered alum little by little. Then add opium.

Remove the iron pan from the fire and put the medicine in a mortar and pestle it for about an hour.

Useful in blepharitis, conjunctivitis, granular lids.

## PATENT MEDICINES OF DR. AGARWAL'S EYE INSTITUTE

RESOLVENT 200 & 500—In all cases of defective eye sight, dull and weak eyes, retinal diseases, cataract, glaucoma,

floating specks, myopia, hypermetropia, astigmatism etc.
Avoid when inflammation or much redness in the eye.

These medicines improve blood circulation. The base is honey, hence it is easily dissolved in the eye.

OPACITOX—It is irritant to the eye and helps to dissolve the foreign matter. Useful in opacity cornea, early cataract, trachoma, chronic conjunctivitis, silent glaucoma.

ELIXIR OCULOSE—It gives cooling sensation. Very useful when there is feeling of heat or burning in the eye, spring catarrh, inflammatory conditions of the eye. It is in the form of surma.

ELIXIR SPECIAL—This surma is black in colour and is very useful when there is watering from the eye or lids stick in the morning, in blepharitis, in weak eyes, also to improve the beauty of the eyes.

OPHTHALMO—It is an eye wash, to be mixed in water about 5 to 20 drops of this lotion to be added in an eye cup. Its action is to tone the tissues and act as an antiseptic.

SOLLUX—It is a very soothing eye drop. Very useful to relieve the strain, feeling of heat or burning sensation, inflammatory conditions, weak eyes.

EYEREX—It is a very useful surma for chronic conjunctivitis with mucoid discharge, trachoma.

OCULO-COOLEX—It is an oil for head massage to refresh the brain or in headache when there is an uncomfortable feeling due to heat. Before applying the oil put a little water on the hairs and massage the head then with this oil for about 10 minutes while the eyes are kept closed.

OCULO-VIGOR—It is a mild laxative made of herbs. It improves digestion and relieves constipation. Very useful in glaucoma, retinal diseases. It is taken by mouth with water or milk.

CENTOFIX—This is in the form of tablets. Usually taken with fruit juice or lemon in water, or with Karela juice and water. This stimulates the action of liver and helps in purifying blood and improve blood circulation.

V-30—It is powder and is used for vapour bath to the eye. Put a pinch in boiling water or in a thermos and take the vapour.

ICINE—These are tablets. It is a tonic to the nervous system and brain. One tablet may be taken daily or on alternate days with a cup of milk or fruit juice.

TRIPHALA GHRITA is an Ayurvedic Preparation of Triphala and clarified butter.

## Homoeopathic Remedies

It is the healing energy which cures a disease. This energy is already present in the body and many diseases and many patients are cured without any treatment. When the energy is not active or is insufficient to fight a disease, remedies are to be used. The action of Homeopathic medicines is to stimulate the dormant energy in the body in a subtle form to cure a disease. Their usefulness depends on the person who prescribes and also on the effectivity of the medicine. If the physician has a primary good intention of healing a patient and is able to transmit his thought power through the medicine, the action of the medicine will be very effective. Right selection of the medicine is also needed. To become a successful Homeopath intuition helps much more than the intellectual knowledge.

## Their Use

1. Usually medicines of 200 potency in globules are used for eye troubles.

2. Better take the medicine in empty stomach once a day or once a week. Dose is about 5 globules.

3. Along with the medicine seek the aid of other methods also so as to bring quick relief as the action of homeopathic remedies is limited and uncertain though they surprise the doctor and the patient at times by remarkable results.

4. When the trouble is connected with the general system of the body their use is more effective.

5. When there is too much accumulation of toxic matter in the system, better clear it up first by enema, purgative, nasal drop etc.

## Medicines

ACONITE—In the first stage of acute inflammatory conditions accompanied by restlessness as acute conjunctivitis, acute iritis, acute glaucoma, stye etc.

ARNICA—In injuries and to check bleeding.

ARSENIC—In mental weakness and general debility.

BELLADONNA—In later stage of acute inflammatory conditions of the eye, headache due to heat or inflammation of the eye.

BRYONIA—In dryness of mucous membrane as Vataja conjunctivitis, feeling of dryness in the eye, Xerosis.

CAUSTICUM—In tumours and warts of the lids.

GELSIMIUM—In stiffness of the muscles of the eye, high tension of the eye and glaucoma.

HEMAMELIS—To prevent bleeding and to absorb bleeding as in vitreous haemorrhage, retinal haemorrhage.

HEPAR SULPH—To prevent suppuration as in ulcer cornea, inflammatory condition of the eye and lid, dacryocystitis.

LYCOPODIUM—In mental weakness and night blindness.

MERC. SOL—Feeling of cold in head and eye, Catarrhal conjunctivitis, iritis, keratitis, erruptions of lids.

NATRUM MUR—In watering of the eye.

NATRUM SULPH—In oedema of the lids and conjunctiva.

NUX VOMICA—In visual disturbances due to digestive disorders. Usually this medicine is taken at bed time.

PHOSPHORIC ACID—In mental weakness, headache, visual defects, diseases of the retina and optic nerve.

PULSATILLA—In Ch. conjunctivitis and coryza where discharge is thick, blepharitis.

PSORINUM—When ulcers slow to heal and in itching skin diseases.

SILICIA—When there is suppuration as in suppurative conjunctivitis, ulcer cornea, chronic dacryocystitis.

SULPHUR—In skin diseases as in erruptions of the lids, blepharitis, frequent styes.

THUJA—In catarrh of the nose and the eye.

## Massage

Massage of the whole body, especially of the head, improves blood circulation and produces relaxation. The top of the head is massaged by rapid, gentle and light rubbing movement of the fingers. Some hair oil or Occulo Coolex may be used for massage. Occulo Coolex may be prepared by mixing about five grains of menthol in one ounce of sweet oil. While the head is massaged, the eyes are to be kept closed. It is good to apply a little water on the head before the application of the oil. The forehead may also be massaged at the same time. Usually seven to ten minutes are sufficient for the massage of the head.

In forehead massage move your body gently from side to side and keep the eyes closed. Place the tips of the fingers lightly on the forehead and allow the forehead to move freely beneath the fingers. When successful, the fingers appear to move in the opposite direction. It is good to get the massage done by someone else.

Massage of the head and the forehead relieves the strain and proves very efficacious in relieving headache and pain in and around the eyeballs.

### Vapour Bath

Vapour bath is a good method to relieve the spasm of the muscles to absorb the blood in haemorrhages, and to improve the blood circulation. The process is as follows:

(a) Take an electric kettle or a bronchitis kettle or a jug containing some water. Let the water boil. One or two crystals of menthol may be added to the boiling water.

(b) Sit before the vapour, and cover the head and the kettle with a thick cloth so that the vapour may not pass out. Take the vapour on the face. While taking the vapour bath breathe deeply and blink frequently. Take the vapour bath till perspiration comes out.

(c) After the vapour bath wipe out the perspiration and put cold pads on the eyes or wash the face with cold water. The water may be splashed against the eyes and face, or the face may be dipped several times in a basin full of water.

## RELAXATION METHODS

We have studied that loss of central fixation is invariably found in all eye troubles. Therefore, any method which improves central fixation will be helpful in curing the eye troubles. The aim of all the relaxation methods is to teach the eye and the mind how to improve central fixation without an effort to see.

### 1. Central Fixation

By central fixation is meant the ability of the eye to look directly at a point, and while doing so to see best with the centre of the sight in the retina. The letter regarded is seen better than the rest of the letters. When the top of a small letter of the Snellen test card at ten or twenty feet is regarded by central fixation, the bottom of the same letter appears less black, but the whole letter is clearer, the black appears a darker shade of black, and the white part of the letter appears whiter. The eyes feel no strain.

When the ability of the eye to see the point regarded best is suppressed partially or completely, the condition is called eccentric fixation. The vision for letters or words is always less distinct than with central fixation. The edges of the letters are not clean cut and have a fuzzy or shadowy margin. The size of letters is altered: they appear larger or smaller than with normal vision. Their shape is distorted; a square letter may seem to be round. Floating specks may occur. Two or more images of one letter may be seen. Pain, fatigue, tension, or discomfort of some kind is usually felt in the eyes during eccentric fixation.

The following procedures are recommended for obtaining central fixation. The patient is told to look at a light at twenty feet or greater distance, then to look a foot or further to one side of the light until it appears less bright. By practice and by increasing or lessening the distance of the point fixed to one side, the patient may soon become convinced that the light is seen best by looking straight at it.

To improve central fixation it is necessary to take the help of a Snellen test card. Take the card in your hand. Keep your sight just below the letter 'C' on the white background. While keeping the sight below the letter, whole of 'C' is visible but the bottom part of 'C' appears more distinct than the top part of 'C'. Now shift your sight to the whole background just above 'C' and note that the top part of 'C' has become more distinct than the bottom part of 'C'. In this way shift your sight three times from bottom to top and top to bottom of 'C'. Similarly practise on the smaller letters up to the sixth or seventh line of the Snellen test card. If the part of the letter regarded does not appear best, close the eyes for half a minute and remember the black or white colour, then open the eyes and practise on the letter. Then increase the distance of Snellen test card to 2,3,4,5,6,7,8,9,10 feet gradually and practise central fixation. While practising central fixation palming may be done at times. If you find difficulty in regarding one part of a letter best, regard one letter of a line in such a manner that the one following it appears less distinct.

To improve central fixation on the reading matter of the book, keep the sight just below the line of letters and shift the sight from one end of the white line to the other. Note that each word coming nearer the sight appears more distinct than the others. Blink gently.

## 2. Palming

All the relaxation methods are simply different ways of relieving the strain, and most patients, though by no means all find palming as the easiest method of relaxation. In palming when the eyes are closed and covered with the palms avoiding pressure on the eyeballs, one sees a black field before the eyes; but when the eyes are diseased or the mind and eyes are under strain, patients fail to see black, but see other colours. Such patients are greatly helped by the memory of a black object—black velvet, silk, ink, letters on the Snellen test card, cap, curtain etc. A familiar black object can often be remembered more easily by the patient than those that are less so. A dressmaker for instance, was able to remember a thread of black silk when she could not remember any other black object. The patient is directed to look at such an object at the distance at which the colour can be seen best, and then to close the eyes and remember the colour. He repeats until the memory appears to be equal to the sight. Then the patient is instructed to cover the closed eyes with the palms of the hands in the manner just described. If the memory of the black is perfect, the whole background will be black. If it is not, or if it does not become so in the course of a few seconds, the eyes are opened and the black object regarded again.

The longer some people palm, the greater the relaxation they obtain and the darker the shade of black they are able both to remember and see black. Others are able to palm successfully for short periods, but begin to strain if they keep it up too long.

## 3. Shifting and Swinging

The normal eye has normal sight when it is at rest. It is at rest or relaxed, when it is moving to prevent stare, strain, or effort to see. Shifting or moving the eyes from side to side with a corresponding movement of the head improves the sight when done properly. It is done wrongly when the eyes move in a different direction from the movement of the head; while turning the head to the right, the eyes turn to the left. Cases have been observed where one or both eyes appear stationary while the head may be moving. In some cases the eyes would move irregularly and unconsciously a longer or shorter distance than the movements of the head.

When the eyes and head move from side to side or in other directions, stationary objects appear to move in the opposite direction. This illusion or the apparent movement of the objects is called swinging. Like many things, the swing can be done wrongly as well as rightly. To be able to practise the swing rightly is a great help to the eyes. The patient can stand beside his table while moving the body, head and eyes from side to side. He can notice that the table and other things in front of him are moving in the direction opposite to the movement of his body. When he looks out of the window, the curtain cord, the vertical bars and other parts of the window will appear to move in the opposite direction, while more distant objects, buildings or trees will appear to move in the same direction as he moves. While walking straight ahead, one can notice that the floor appears to move towards him. If the patient is conscious of the movement of the floor and other objects, the stare and strain is prevented, and the vision is always improved; but if he does not notice the movement of objects when he himself moves, he is apt to strain.

Some people have difficulty in imagining any stationary object to be moving. They feel absolutely certain that the stationary object is always stationary and cannot be expected to move when the body sways from side to side in a long or short movement. It is absolutely necessary that all persons with imperfect sight should become able to imagine stationary objects to be moving. A very successful method of teaching nervous people how to imagine stationary objects to be moving is as follows:

The Snellen test card is fastened to a support about fifteen feet away from the patient. When the patient looks at a point about three feet to the right of the test card, the card is to the left of the point regarded, and advances further to the left when the point regarded is moved to the right. When the patient is directed to regard a point to the left of the Snellen test card, the card moves to the right side of the point regarded.

The greater the shift from one point to another, the wider becomes the swing. By repetition, the patient becomes able to realize that whenever a point regarded is to the right of the card, the card and all other objects are to the left of the point regarded. When the eyes move to one side of the card, the card moves to the opposite side and this movement of the card can always be demonstrated.

This method is always a truth without any exceptions because no matter how much the patient may insist that he is right, he has to acknowledge that when he looks to the right, the Snellen test card moves to the left and this movement is so decided that it very soon becomes impossible for the patient to fail to imagine stationary objects to be moving whenever the eyes move from right to left, or from left to right, or in any other direction. This demonstraion may be made very convincing with a little time and patience.

The shorter the swing, the greater the benefit to the eyes; but it is interesting to observe that swinging the head and eyes a long distance from side to side is more easily accomplished than a short movement. Swinging can be practised both with the eyes open and closed.

## Long Swing

When the shifting of the sight is more than an inch, it is called long swing. Long swing is useful in relieving eye discomforts and headache, and helps to adopt a short swing by shortening the long movement.

## Short Swing

When the shifting of the sight is less than an inch it is called short swing. Short swing improves the vision.

## 4. Mental Pictures

The mind is busy as long as we are awake. We remember many things and are consciously or unconsciously shifting from one thing to another. Those things that we remember or imagine mentally are called mental pictures.

Mental pictures are very important. For example, if a patient can remember and imagine a black letter or other object perfectly with the eyes closed and with the eyes open, the patient has a normal eye with normal sight; but if the same patient remembers or imagines a letter or other object imperfectly, the vision becomes imperfect, a change takes place in the normal shape of the eyeball and the eye becomes imperfect—too long, too short, or of an irregular shape.

Imperfect memory increases the hardness of the eyeball and produces other disagreeable symptoms and pain.

To obtain perfect mental pictures requires a perfect relaxation. If the patient can see at the near point a small letter 'O' with a white centre whiter than it really is, or whiter than the rest of the white card, it is usually possible to close the eyes and remember or imagine a perfect mental picture of the letter.

To many patients the memory of a small black dot is the best mental picture. When the mental picture of a dot is perfect, the dot appears to move with a slow, short, easy swing. Any effort to remember or imagine the dot impairs the mental picture. The vision of a perfectly black dot may be used to improve the vision of large letters or other objects. By practice, one becomes able to remember or imagine a perfect dot at all times and in all places when desired. The memory of a black dot is beneficial also in other ways. When the eyes are tired, the perfect memory of a dot at once brings a feeling of perfect rest. Symptoms of various diseases of the eye have been relieved at once by the memory of a perfect dot.

To some patients mental picture of a black object produces strain while the memory of some pleasant scenery or beautiful colours which are remembered without effort give relaxation. There are certain shades of colours which do produce mental strain and at the same time cause lowering of the vision. Green, no matter what shade of green it may be, is usually a rest and relaxation to the mind and eyes.

## 5. White Line

The white space in between the lines of print is called the white line. If one can imagine a thin white line in this white space below the letters of the test card or beneath a line of fine print, it is very helpful. This thin white line is only imagined, it is not seen, because the line is not really there. It is valuable in the treatment and cure of presbyopia, hypermetropia, astigmatism, many cases of myopia and other eye troubles. One should imagine it in the right way. The wrong way is to try to imagine the thin white line and the black letters at the the same time. This causes a strain which always blurs the black letter and prevents the thin white line from being imagined.

Many patients complain that they have difficulty in imagining the thin white line. To overcome this, one should imagine it just below some word or collection of words which are known. The line is then readily imagined and it can be imagined extending from one side of the page to the other, and wherever it becomes manifest the vision is always improved. One can read rapidly, clearly, and without discomfort, when he is conscious of the thin white line, but to fix the sight on the black letters and expect to read them is a mistake which very few teachers or students have observed. The fact that one cannot read properly when looking at the black letters should be more widely known. Much time has been lost in the classroom by teachers trying to force the children to look directly at the blackness of the black letters. When black letters are regarded and seen best, much pain, discomfort, or imperfect sight is experienced.

One cannot be sure when imagining the thin white line that the eyes are directed towards it. When one plans to look at the thin white line and while trying to read something feels discomfort or pain, it means that the eyes are not directed on the thin white line as the reader may imagine.

If the patient cannot imagine the white line easily, he is told to close his eyes and think of a series of white objects:

he may recall a white-washed wall, a white cow or bull, or a pot of white paint. He is then directed to open his eyes again and look at the white spaces, imagining them to be as white as the white objects he remembered. He is told to close his eyes again and imagine that he has a pot of white paint and and a fine pen and that he is drawing a thin white line beneath a line of print, then to open his eyes and imagine that he is drawing a white line beneath each line of letters on the fundamental card as he moves his head from side to side. He is told to blink as he shifts from one end of the line to the other, to occasionally look away and to close his eyes frequently for half a minute or so to rest them.

By practising in this way, letters which could not be seen before appear black and distinct. As one's ability to read is improved, the card is brought closer and the patient is instructed to practise in this way, until the entire card can be read at six inches from his eyes.

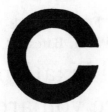

50 FEET

**C**

30 FEET

**R B**

20 FEET

**T F P**

15 FEET

**5 C G O**

10 FEET

**4 K B E R**

5 FEET

**3 V Y F P T**

4 FEET

**2 Q C O G D □ C**

3 FEET

**R Z 3 B 8 S H K F O**

Snellen Test Card — Pocket Size

Fundamentals
By W. H. Bates, M. D.

# 1. Central Fixation is seeing best where you are looking.

2. Favourable conditions: Light may be bright or dim. The distance of the print from the eyes, where seen best, also varies with people.

3. Shifting: With normal sight the eyes are moving all the time.

4. Swinging: When the eyes move slowly or rapidly from side to side, stationary objects appear to move in the opposite direction.

5. Long Swing: Stand with the feet about one foot apart, turn the body to the right—at the same time lifting the heel of the left foot. Do not move the head or eyes or pay any attention to the apparent movement of stationary objects. Now place the left heel on the floor, turn the body to the left, raising the heel of the right foot. Alternate.

6. Drifting Swing: When practising this swing, one pays no attention to the clearness of stationary objects, which appear to be moving. The eyes wander from point to point slowly, easily, or lazily, so that the stare or strain may be avoided.

7. Variable Swing: Hold the forefinger of one hand six inches from the right eye and about the same distance to the right, look straight ahead and move the head a short distance from side to side. The finger appears to move.

8. Stationary Objects Moving: By moving the head and eyes a short distance from side to side, being sure to blink, one can imagine stationary objects to be moving.

9. Memory: Improving the memory of letters and other objects improves the vision for everything.

10. Imagination: We see only what we think we see, or what we imagine. We can only imagine what we remember.

11. Rest: All cases of imperfect sight are improved by closing the eyes and resting them.

12. Palming: The closed eyes may be covered with the palm of one or both hands.

13. Blinking: The normal eye blinks or closes and opens very frequently.

14. Mental Pictures: As long as one is awake one has all kinds of memories of mental pictures. If these pictures are remembered easily, perfectly, the vision is benefited.

# Chapter XII

## REFRACTION AND DISEASES

### Normal Eye

1. The normal eye reads twenty feet line on the Snellen test card at 20ft. distance quite clearly without any effort and the vision is recorded $^{20}/_{20}$. The letters are perfectly black and distinct. In reading, fine print is distinctly visible at 12 inches.

*How to test the vision.* Distant vision (D.V.). Place the Snellen test card at 20 feet or 6 metres distance in good light. Read the chart with each eye separately and both eyes together; cover one eye with the palm of one hand avoiding any pressure on the eyeball. The vision is expressed by a fraction, the numerator of which corresponds to the number of feet separating the patient from the chart, and the denominator to the number written on the line read. If the sight is normal, the vision will be $^{20}/_{20}$ or $^{6}/_{6}$; if from 20 feet one reads 50 feet line the vision will be $^{20}/_{50}$.

To test the near vision take the Snellen reading test type or Fundamentals. Test the sight at 12 inches, also at nearer to longer distance. Write the number of reading test type or Fundamentals read at so many inches, e.g. Fundamentals No. 8 at 12 inches.

2. Another test—To the normal eye a black letter appears as black at the distance as at the near, while to the defective eye there is a change in the shade of black.

3. While looking through a pin-hole the vision of the normal eye is decreased while that of the imperfect eye is improved.

4. The normal eye is quiet and at rest, feels no fatigue, pain

or strain while the defective eye gets tired, feels pain or strain. Headache is quite common in defective eye patients.

5. The use of atropine for the examination of the eye is generally harmful and its use for such purposes should be avoided as far as possible.

## Myopia

Myopia or short sightedness is an error of refraction. The sight is usually very good at about ten inches or nearer while very dim or blurred for objects at ten feet or farther. The eyeball is elongated and the eye cannot focus for distant objects. By putting concave lens before the eye the distant objects appear clear.

The cause of myopia is staring or an effort to see distant objects. Look at the eye chart at 20 ft. Stare at the top letter and observe the sight for smaller letters has become dim. Now strain at 12 inches on fine print in dim light and observe that the sight for distance has improved.

### Treatment

1. Learn correct blinking and keep the eyes half open without squeezing or screwing.

2. Learn central fixation on ૩ૐ chart and Snellen eye chart at 1 to 5 ft.

3. Read fine print in dim light and read the eye chart at 10 to 20 ft. in good light with gentle blinking.

4. Frequent palming and reading distant chart.

5. Avoid an effort to see distant objects.

6. Learn the art of seeing a view card.

7. Observe side objects moving while walking or driving.

8. Nourishing diet if patient mentally or physically weak. (Study *Mind and Vision* or *Yoga of Perfect Sight*)...

MYOPIA IN SCHOOLS—To prevent and cure myopia in schools place the Snellen test card on the wall of each class room, and every day the children should read it from their seats, silently, with both eyes and with each eye. In one week's time many children will show improvement in their sight.

## Hypermetropia

In hypermetropia or long sightedness the distant sight is usually better than the reading sight. The eyeball is flattened. Usually hypermetropia is the cause of headache, pain, fatigue and other discomforts of the eye. Convex or plus lenses counteract the condition of hypermetropia.

The cause of hypermetropia is strain at the near point. Rest and relaxation when properly employed cures hypermetropia and other discomforts. Cases who do not respond well to the treatment may be helped with glasses along with relaxation treatment.

1. Read Fundamentals or fine print daily in good light and dim light without or with glasses.

2. Shift sight on the white lines just below the lines of letters.

3. Place the chart at about 20ft. distance in dim light and hold the Fundamental chart in hand in good light. Read the distant chart and Fundamental chart alternately.

4. Look at the blank surface as sky, grass, wall and read the Fundamental chart in hand alternately.

5. Seeing cinema, moon, kite, trees, birds flying are very helpful.

## Astigmatism

Astigmatism is always accompanied with myopia or hypermetropia. Letters on the chart may appear distorted and
patient frequently makes mistakes in reading the letters of the
chart. Many cases complain of difficulty in reading and
headache.

Learn gentle blinking and keep the upper lids down.
Exercises given to benefit myopia or hypermetropia prove
very helpful. For details study *Mind and Vision* and *Yoga
of Perfect Sight*.

## Presbyopia or Old Age Sight

Persons nearing about forty and upwards have difficulty
in reading books or news papers, especially at night, although
their distant sight may be normal. They are usually depen-
dent upon their glasses for reading. This condition has been
called old age sight or presbyopia.

The decline of reading sight is regular in most cases and
one can judge the approximate age from man's glasses. For
example, at the age of forty one will require plus one, at the
age of fifty plus two, at the age of sixty plus three. Generally
presbyopia comes early in hypermetropic eye, and late in the
myopic eye.

The cause of decline in sight is strain which chiefly affects
the near vision. In some cases the condition goes on getting
worse and frequently glasses are changed, till no glasses fit
the eyes.

Reading of fine print daily in good light and dim light from
the age of thirty five prevents the advent of presbyopia. When
presbyopia has affected the eyes, reading fine print or Funda-

mental card without or with glasses is very helpful. In some cases a change occurs after fifty and sight begins to return and the number of glasses goes on reducing. At this time a little relaxation treatment and reading fine print become an immense aid. The sight varies due to variation in health and action of liver; so in old age sweets and fat should be lessened and bitter and green leafy vegetables may be added in diet. Application of honey or Resolvent in the eyes along with sun treatment for about two minutes give vigor to the eyes and improve the sensitiveness of the retina.

## Treatment of Eye Diseases

### Diseases of Eye Lid

BLEPHARITIS—Clean the lid margins and expose to the rays of the sun, apply Elixir special or Eyerex, Penicilin ointment. HOMEOPATHY—Sulphur 200 or Merc. Sol. 200 once a week.

STYE—In the early stage vapour, rubbing finger or gold ring and touch the stye frequently. Vapour liquifies the hardness while touching with finger or gold creates a vibration to increase the vitality of the cells. Frequent palming.
Hom.—Heparsulph. 200.

TRICHIASIS—Remove inverted hairs by cilia forceps. If necessary operation of the lid.

TRACHOMA—Opacitox, Eyerex, sun, Sulphanomide ointment, Aureomycin ointment.

DACRYOCYSTITIS—Lacrymal sac is diseased and obstructed.

Pus comes out on pressure, watering.

Treat. Remove the pus by pressure frequently and drop Penicilin lotion or Antiseptic lotion or apply Elixir Oculose. Syringing with Penicilin lotion.

Nasal douche or Sharbindo oil in the nose.

Karela juice with Centofix tablet by mouth.

Hom. Silicia or Heparsulph 200 once a week.

## Diseases of Conjunctiva

SIMPLE CONJUNCTIVITIS—Slight redness, mucoid discharge, gluing of lids in the morning.

Treat—Wash with Ophthalmo or Triphala lotion or saline.

Apply Eyerex, Elixir Special, some ointment at bed time. Oculo-Vigor by mouth.

ACUTE CONJUNCTIVITIS—Red eye, thick discharge, lids inflamed.

Treat—Wash the eye and drop mercurochrome lotion, Argyrol, Protargol, Penicilin, Zinc and alum drops. Terramycin ointment at bed time.

Purgative and adjust diet. Avoid hot things as chillies etc.

PTERYGIUM—A fold extending from conjunctiva to cornea. This can be prevented by the application of Eyerex or Elixir Oculose. Advise operation when sufficiently extends on the cornea.

OPHTHALMIA—When whole eyeball under inflammation as in acute iritis or acute glaucoma. Pain, much watering, glare, copper coloured redness.

Treat—Vapour and nasal drops. Strong enema or Brooklax. Dry diet, reduce water in drinking, no milk or its preparations. Soothing drops as Sollux, Elixir. Sun and vapour. No irritant medicines to be applied in the eye.

## Diseases of Cornea

KERATITIS—Inflammation of cornea and formation of blood vessels.

Treat—Vapour or fomentation, sun, soothing medicines. Cortisone, Penicilin drops. Sharbindo oil in the nose. Motions to be kept clear. Diet regulated.

ULCER CORNEA—Same as for Keratitis.

OPACITY CORNEA—Opacitox, Resolvent with open eye sun treatment. When opacity very dense as after small pox then usually no treatment helps.

Arcus Senilis—A white ring around the cornea is formed usually in old age. It is not harmful and no treatment is required. Apply Resolvent and give sun treatment to improve the health of the eye.

KERATOCONUS—Bulging of cornea without any inflammation. Keep eyes half open and blink frequently, relaxation by frequent palming. Contact lenses.

## CATARACT

MATURE cataract needs operation. In the early stage opacitox, Resolvent and reading Fundamentals in the good and dim light are very helpful. Long sun treatment is usually avoided.

Some cases have little cataract but the vision is greatly reduced in comparison to the formation of cataract. Such cases are usually under great eye strain and treatment ought to be tried instead of telling them to wait for operation.

If there is no perception of light to the patient, the case is not fit for operation.

Degenerative cataract develops quickly and operation is the right thing. Cataract due to strain as in high myopia or hypermetropia develops very slow and needs relaxation treatment. After operation the patient needs glasses.

## GLAUCOMA

DIMNESS in vision, pain and strain, headache, halo around light, nasal field contracted, pupil dilated, tension high. Symptoms vary too much in glaucoma cases but high tension is a very common symptom.

Treat—Vapour, Sharbindo oil in the nose  Oculo-vigor at bed time, Sun and relaxation treatment, diet laxative. Operation is usually not beneficial.

Hom. Gelsimium 200

In absolute glaucoma no benefit is possible.

## NIGHT BLINDNESS

NIGHT blindness since birth is not curable. Such cases have good vision in light and no organic defect in the retina is visible.

Night blindness due to deficiency of Vitamin A or due to strain can be benefited.

Treat—Triphala ghrita, Vitamin A, green vegetables, carrot etc., Sun, Resolvent. Head massage. Mild purgative as

Oculo-Vigor daily at bed time if bowels constipated. Liver extract or fried liver by mouth. Teach the patient how to walk in dim light. He should shift the sight with his steps and not stare at any object.

## QUESTIONS AND ANSWERS

*Q: Often, when I am trying to see a thing, it becomes clear at first, then when I blink it fades away. What should I do to overcome it?*

A: Blinking can be done correctly, and it can be done incorrectly. You strain while you blink. The normal eye blinks easily and frequently. Strain is always accompanied by the stare. By standing and swaying from side to side so that your whole body, head, and eyes move together, the stare is lessened.

*Q: What causes redness and smarting sensation of the eye even when plenty of sun treatment has been given? Should one continue with sun treatment under the circumstances?*

A: Take the sun treatment frequently for about five minutes at a time daily, increasing the length of time until the eyes become accustomed to the sun. The eyes should always be benefited after the sun treatment, and one should always feel relaxed. When done properly, the redness and smarting should soon disappear. If the eyes are not benefited, it is an indication that you strain while taking the treatment. Alternate the sun treatment with palming or closing the eyes to rest them.

*Q: Is resting the eyes by palming a more effective cure for smarting of the eyes than the sun treatment?*

A: This depends upon the individual. Some are benefited

more by palming, while others receive more benefit from the sun treatment.

*Q: Why is it that I have perfect vision only in flashes?*
A: You have not yet lost your unconscious habit of straining. When relaxation methods are practised faithfully at all times, the flashes of improved vision become more frequent and last longer until the vision becomes continuously good.

*Q: What causes twitching of the eyelids?*
A: Strain causes twitching of the eyelids and this is relieved by rest and relaxation. Palming, sun treatment, swinging, concentration on candle flame and blinking are very beneficial.

*Q: I have bad eyesight due to some retinal disorder. Can my eyes be benefited?*
A: Yes, relaxation methods can greatly help you. (Study Mind & Vision)

*Q: What is best to prevent cataract?*
A:   1. Apply Resolvent 200 in the eyes.
     2. Concentrate on a candle flame while counting 100 respirations.
     3. Read fine print in good light and candle light with or without glasses.

*Q: I am presbyopic and use glasses of plus 2.5 for reading. When I go to a hill station, my eyesight is improved and I read news paper without glasses. Can you explain this fact?*
A: Looking at the greens and seeing the things moving in the opposite direction while climbing up produces relaxation in the eye muscles, hence the sight is improved. Strain is the

cause of your defective vision while relaxation is the proof of your improved vision.

*Q: Why do you recommend reading in dim light for a myopic patient?*

A: Strain of reading in dim light causes hypermetropia, so it becomes helpful in myopic patients. After reading some small print in dim light for sufficient time with a little strain brings definite improvement in the distant vision of a myopic patient.

*Q: You recommend reading fine print in dim light and close to the eyes, but these ideas are quite opposite to the orthodox belief. How do you justify your standpoint?*

A: Those who advise you to read big print in good light at a long distance are your parents and teachers and doctors, they are mostly above forty, and at this age they lose the faculty of reading small print in dim light and at a near point. What suits them, they advise to others also. But for young and children reading fine print in candle light is extremely beneficial. You can test for yourself whether you read better in bright electric light or in candle light.

*Q: I am hypermetropic. What do you advise for me?*

A: Place the Snellen Eye Testing Chart at 15 ft. distance in dim light. Hold the Fundamental chart to read in good light. Make an effort to read the distant chart, then shift your sight on the white lines of the Fundamentals with gentle blinking. Alternate. Strain at a distance will lessen the hypermetropia and finally make the eye normal.

*Q: My daughter is four years old, she has developed squint and her right eye turns towards the nose.*

A: Young children can usually be cured of squint by the use of atropine. A one percent solution is dropped into the better eye or both eyes daily for about one year. The atropine makes it more difficult for the child to see, and makes the sunlight disagreeable. In order to overcome this difficulty the child has to relax the eye muscles, and the relaxation cures the squint. Swaying the child in a circle is also very useful.

Q: I use glasses for reading only and am fifty years old. Without glasses I cannot work. Now these glasses do not give clear vision. What to do?

A: Concentrate on a candle flame while counting one hundred respirations. Read small print with glasses in good light and in candle light.

Q: I have discarded glasses and I ride considerably on cycle, often I go on a trip in the car and after every trip I find my eyes stronger. This, I think, is due to the rapid changing of focus in viewing scenery going by so fast.

A: The rapid motion compels rapid shifting and helps in relieving the strain.

Q: Every year I get inflammation in my eyes, the glare troubles me and I use dark glasses. Can my eyes be benefited?

A: Take sun treatment for a few minutes daily. At night practise concentration on a candle flame and read fine print.

Q: When I travel in a bus, my eyes are greatly strained.

A: Imagine side objects moving backwards, do not stare at any object. Better look at the movements of the conductor or read something so as to avoid the habit of staring.

*Q: What is most helpful when one is highly myopic and finds it almost impossible to see without glasses?*

A: Practise palming frequently and read fine print with gentle blinking in dim light.

*Q: Why is fine print beneficial?*

A: Fine print is beneficial because it cannot be read by a strain or effort, the eyes must be relaxed.

*Q: How can I correct the vision of my three-year-old son, who won't palm and does not understand it? He is far-sighted.*

A: Make a test card with black letters on white paper. The letters are to be composed of E's pointing in various directions. These E's are to be graduated in size, from about $3\frac{1}{2}$ inches to a quarter of an inch. Let the child read them from 10 to 20 feet away. Have him blink constantly while telling in which direction the E's are pointing.

*Q: I have improved my sight by palming, but when I read for any length of time, the pain returns.*

A: When you read and your eyes pain you, it means that you are straining your eyes. More frequent palming and reading fine print with gentle blinking will help you.

*Q: Is it all right to palm while lying down? Is it better to sit or stand while doing so? If the arms get tired is it all right to rest the elbows on a desk or something like that while palming. Or is it best to hold the elbows up free from all support?*

A: It is all right to palm while lying down. Palming should not be done while one is standing. The elbows should rest on a desk or on a cushion placed in the lap. One should be in as comfortable a position as possible while palming, in order to obtain the most benefit.

*Q: If type can be seen more distinctly with the eyes partly closed, is it advisable to read that way?*

A: No, it is not advisable to read that way because it is a strain, and alters the shape of the eyeball.

## NURSING OF THE EYE

**1. Eyelids:**—Upper eye lids to be kept downwards to keep the eyes less open without screwing or squeezing or straining. Wide open eyes usually increase the strain as we often see in cases of myopia or glaucoma.

Look at a letter on the Snellen test card at ten feet or more with wide open eyes by lowering the chin and raising the lids, and observe that the vision is lowered.

To get the right habit of the lids keep the lids down consciously and blink frequently. Frequent palming and swinging and bandaging help to gain the right habit.

Walk with lids down and blink at each step. Count one, two, three, four. At four raise the chin and glance at the distance.

Take a ball and throw it up about one foot high and shift the head and eyes with lids down with the movement of the ball.

**2. Blinking:**— In blinking the upper lids come a little down and then again raised. It is a short and gentle movement of the lids. In winking the upper lid touches the lower lid with a jerk. Blinking is good and normal while winking is abnormal and harmful. Educate the lids to blink gently.

a. Take a mirror, look at one eye and blink, look at the other eye and blink. Palm at intervals.

b. Take a ball and shift it from hand to hand and blink.

c. Walk and blink at each step. Observe that the side objects appear to move backwards.

**3. Movements of The Eyeball:**—The eyes should always move with the movement of the head. Keeping the head fixed and moving the eyes in various directions causes strain. Or moving the head in one direction and moving the eyes in the opposite direction greatly increases the strain.

a. Look to the right and look to the left with the movement of the head. Try in a wrong way also and observe that the strain begins to manifest.

b. Move the body, head and eyes like a pendulum with eyes closed. Observe that the eyeballs also move with the movement of the head. This movement is also visible to the observer from outside.

c. Walk like an elephant with a sway. Put the right step and sway the body head and eyes to the right and vice versa.

d. Take a book and hold it at a distance where the print is seen best and read it while shifting the head and eyes a little from side to side.

**4. Reading:**—To relieve the discomforts while reading the following methods are very helpful:

a. Read fine print in good light and candle light alternately with gentle blinking.

b. Shift the sight just below the line of letters on the white space in between the lines of print and blink at each line.

c. Sway the body forward and backward and read.

d. Read fine print and some book alternately.

**5. Travelling:**—While travelling in a train or a motarcar observe that the side objects appear to move backwards. Keeping the gaze fixed on any object causes strain. While marketing avoid to see each and every shop and signboard. Go straight to the required shop and keep up blinking.

**6. Sun Treatment:**—Sun treatment is very beneficial to relieve inflammation of the eyeball and many other discomforts and to improve the vision.

**a. With Eyes Closed:**—Close the eyes and shift the body, head and eyes like a pendulum from side to side. This shifting keeps relaxation. If the sun is hot, cover the head with a napkin.

**b. Sun Treatment for Babies**—Hold the baby in such a way that the sun rays fall on the face. Then sway the baby with gentle movement.

**c. Sun Treatment Below a Tree**—If the sun is hot or the patient very sensitive to light, then stand below a tree with eyes closed and sway while facing the sun.

## EYE WASH—EYE DROP—EYE APPLICATION

**Eye Wash**

*Splashing*—Splash cold water or warm water with the hand in a gentle way.

*Eye cup*—Fill the eye cup with water and place the lower margin of the cup against the lower eye lid. Upper margin of the cup remains free. Keep the sight downwards and blink frequently. Saline or Ophthalmo may also be used for eye wash.

*Eye wash in a basin*—Fill the basin with water. Dip the face in water and have a short sway of the face in the water with gentle blinking. Take the face out for breathing. Repeat 10 to 20 times. A tea spoon of salt may be added in the water.

## Eye Drops

Hold the dropper in such a way that the eye lotion does not enter into its rubber and drop the lotion in the outer part of the eye.

## Application

Take the required quantity of the medicine at the ends of the rod and apply it gently in the eye while lowering the lower eye lid with the thumb. For the right eye use left hand, for the left eye use right hand to hold the rod.

## PALMING EDUCATION

WHEN the eyes are tired, closing the eyes for a moment clears the vision and a kind of relief is felt in the eyes. But as some light still comes through the closed eyelids, a still greater relief can be obtained by excluding this light as well. This is done by covering the closed eyes with the palms of the hands in such a way as to avoid pressure on the eyeballs. This practice is called 'PALMING'. When the eyes with normal sight are closed and covered so as to shut all the light, the retina of the eye does not receive any light and the result is that one sees or experiences perfect black. Palming is one of the best methods for relieving strain and securing relaxation to improve eyesight.

While palming it is good to imagine something black as a letter of the Snellen eye chart, a piece of black velvet, black paint, a curtain, coaltar etc. For some people it is difficult to recall the memory of black object but they find it easy to recall the memory of pleasant and familiar objects, e.g. a boat floating in a river, a flower, etc. Girls like to imagine their dolls, boys like to imagine a game of cricket or table-tennis, mothers like to imagine the face of their children. When the imagination is perfect according to the reality, one sees perfect dark before the eyes while palming.

Some patients while palming see all sorts of colours but not black. This is due to an effort to imagine or see something. Such patients may try the following method:

Take a piece of black velvet and put it on a cushion which is being used to rest the elbows while doing palming. Look at the black velvet for a second and immediately close the eyes for about half a minute, repeat ten or twenty times till you find that the imagination of black can continue.

Palming may be done for five to ten minutes or more. It is good to palm before going to bed to induce good sleep. When there is a feeling of strain or headache during summer, wash the eyes and face with cold water, dip the hands in cold water and palm for about half an hour. While palming have some cold drink or fruit juice now and then. Cataract patients are greatly benefited by frequent palming.

When palming is successful, it yields wonderful results. I remember a very very interesting case. A boy aged about ten years, son of a merchant, was blind with his right eye since birth although the organ of sight was apparently quite normal. When he was asked to imagine something while palming, he related a perfect experience. "A customer comes to my shop and wants two ounce of butter. My father takes the butter with a spoon and weighs it in the balance. The customer pays money to my father and goes away." The boy was seeing all this mentally as if the thing was going on actually. The result was that his blind eye began to see first big letters and then smaller letters of the eye chart. And it was very joyful and interesting event when the boy gained normal vision in two hours by repeated palming and practice on the chart.

An engineer aged about sixty years was using glasses of $+3$ for about twenty years for reading. It was a surprise to him to improve his sight to read the news paper without glasses in about a month's time. A myopic girl after palming frequently read small print in dim light and improved the distant vision to normal in about two weeks time.

What are the signs of perfect palming?

1. When palming is perfect, the colour of any object remembered is remembered perfectly and one feels perfectly relaxed and one sees a perfect black field before the eyes when they are closed and covered.

2. When the eyes are opened perfect sight comes instantaneously and the letters on the chart are seen perfectly black and are distinctly recognised.

3. The white centres of the letters called halos seem to be whiter than the margin of the chart.

For more details study the book YOGA OF PERFECT SIGHT.

## ART OF SEEING

Treatment by the art of seeing pictures proves greatly helpful in the improvement of eye sight. Select a coloured or black and white view card. Look at the near objects, then at the far objects and set the mind and the eye between near and far objects. Soon the three dimensional character of the objects will begin to manifest and the details will begin to appear. Flatness of the picture initially seen will become three dimensional. Then set yourself in that environment, your mind and eyes will be greatly relaxed. The vision will be found improved. Parctice with one eye separately is easier.

A girl student had bad eyesight, a condition of semi-blindness had manifested. She often suffered from headache and pain in the eyeballs. She could hardly read four lines of the chart from ten feet. With the help of blinking she could read one line more but yet there were three lines more to read. She was given a picture card of Taj Mahal to develop the art of seeing. When the picture appeared three dimensional as if she was actually looking at Tajmahal and its surroundings and trees etc., she exclaimed, "Lovely! beautiful! the sun appears shining on the walls and windows. Every detail of Taj Mahal appears sharply, and my vision is getting improved." When she was asked to read the chart, she could easily read the last line and her vision was recorded normal in fifteen minutes' practice. Since then the child enjoys perfect eyesight.

Another case of hypermetropia of plus four in the left eye was finding it difficult to read the Fundamental card and often got headache in his practice. When he was taught the art of seeing a picture card, the hypermetropic eye began to respond to relax and improved considerably. In three days' practice it began to read fine print and suffered no more from pain and other discomforts.

## TREATMENT OF VISUAL DEFECTS

Three Principles of Treatment:

**1. Elimination**—Educate the patient how to get rid of the habit of staring or making an effort to see by the proper use of the eyes in reading, writing, sewing, seeing cinema, reading the Snellen eye chart etc. Blinking is very important.

**Stimulation**—Improve the blood circulation and sensitiveness of the retina by sun rays, breathing, central fixation exercises, concentration on candle flame, reading fine print in good light and candle light, tonics, massage, etc.

**Relaxation**—Relaxation of the mind and eyes by rest, palming, swinging, memory of a letter or an object, looking at a blank surface, sky or green grass without effort, bandaging, Tarpana treatment, art of seeing pictures.

### Important Points

1. Anything that will rest the mind will benefit the eyes.

2. Temporary benefit comes quickly but for permanent cure time varies with different individuals.

3. Generally persons who had not worn glasses, are benefited more quickly.

4. Glasses should be discarded if good improvement is the aim. When this cannot be done, use of glasses may be permitted for the necessity.

5. Children respond more quickly than adults.

6. All patients can not discard glasses but all can be benefited more or less.

7. Any method which does not bring quick relief should be replaced by another method. The chief aim is to produce relaxation.

## BANDAGE

1. **Cold Pack Bandage**—Soak the cotton pads in cold water and put them on the eyes and bandage for about 15 minutes. It is very soothing to the weak eyes especially after vapour bath.

2. **Potato Bandage**—Take smashed potato and put the paste on the cotton pad and over the paste put a thin piece of cloth or gauze. Then put these potato pads on the eyes and

bandage them for about 15 minutes or more. It is very soothing when there is a feeling of heat in the eyes.

**3. Wheat Flour Bandage**—Take wheat powder and add water to it to make a thick paste. Put the pads on cotton pads and over that put a thing piece of cloth or gauze and bandage the eyes for about half an hour. This greatly helps in minor inflammations of the eye and to relieve the strain.

**4. Ginger Bandage**— Prepare the wheat flour pads as above, then put a thin layer of vaseline over which little dry ginger powder is sprinkled. Put these ginger pads over the eyes and bandage for half to one hour. It is very useful in chronic diseases of the eye.

**5. Mud Bandage**—Like the wheat flour bandage, mud is also applied. It is very useful when there is a feeling of great heat and burning sensation.

**6. Milk Cream Bandage**—Like the wheat flour bandage milk-cream bandage is done to soften the tissues and to relieve the tension. It is especially useful when there is a feeling of dryness in the eyes and when hairs of eyes fall frequently.

**7. Onion Bandage**—Similarly Onion bandage is done. It is beneficial in chronic retinal diseases and in night blindness and in glaucoma.

**8. Tarpana Bandage**—Tarpana is very useful in dull and defective eyes. It gives vigor to the eyes and develops beauty and a sort of glow in the eyes. We have explained Tarpana somewhere else in this book.

## ENEMA

Enema proves very useful in severe inflammatory conditions of the eye and in retinal disorders. Take an enema-can and apply little vaseline or oil at the nozzle. Place the enema-can at about 2 ft height.

**Ordinary Enema**—About one litre of warm water and add to it one tea spoon of salt or lemon juice. Take the enema at bed time or early in the morning once or twice a week.

2. Take an ounce of sterilized sweet oil and put it in the enema-can and let the oil go into the rubber tubing. Then add warm water mixed with salt.

**Strong Enema**—Dissolve about 10 grains of caustic soda in two pints of warm water and put it in the enema-can.

It is very useful when there is acute redness with severe pain in the eyeballs and head. One enema may be sufficient to relieve the congestion of the eye and the tension. After the enema patient may take cold hip-bath or put cold pack on the abdomen for about 20 to 30 minutes. On the enema day the diet should be soft as Khichri, a preparation of rice and pulse.

**Tonic Enema**—Tonic enema is given to increase the vitality and in nervous weakness. First relieve the constipation by an ordinary enema. Then give tonic enema.

Take 4 to 8 ounces of warm milk and add to it one ounce of honey and one ounce of sweet oil. Mix well and give the enema. Retain it for about 15 to 30 minutes. Then go to latrine.

When there is a feeling of dryness in the head and eyes or in cases of optic atrophy and degeneration of retina, tonic enema greatly helps along with relaxation exercises.

**Glycerine Enema**—When children suffer from constipation and redness in the eyes, glycerine enema proves very helpful.

## HIP BATH AND COLD PACK

Cold relieves congestion, reduces heat and burning sensation, tones the tissues and nerves; useful in inflammatory conditions of the eye and in chronic retinal disorders.

**Hip Bath**—Fill the bathtub with cold water so much so that water remains upto the navel when the patient sits in the tub. Keep the legs out. Rub the abdomen with a soft cloth for about 20 minutes. Take hip bath usually after the enema or about an hour before meal.

**Cold Pack**—When hip bath is not convenient, cold pack may be given. Take a wet towel and fold it and put it on the abdomen and cover it with a woollen cloth. Keep the cold pack for about half an hour or more.

## VITAMINS

**Vitamin A**—Vitamin A is very useful in night blindness or when the light adaptation is defective as is usually found in high myopia or in retinal disorders.

It is usually found in yellow coloured vegetables and fruits as carrot, papaya, mango, egg, butter, milk, codliver oil, liver etc.

Medicines rich in Vitamin A—Super D codliver oil, Nestrovit, Abidol, Tirphala Ghirta (Ayurvedic preparation)

**Vitamin B**—as Berin tablets, marmite.

It is useful in inflammatory conditions of retina and cornea, etc.

## HOW TO WRITE A TREATMENT CHART?

1. Divide the cases into 3 catagories—easily curable, curable with difficulty, partially curable.

**Easily Curable**—Ordinary headache, eye strain, low error, patients requiring prevention of error.

Such cases need simple instructions as eye education to

use the eyes in the proper way, palming, blinking, reading Snellen chart, reading fine print. Long programme is avoided.

**Curable With Difficulty**—High error of refraction, early cases of glaucoma or retinal disorder or cataract, floating specks, amblyopia and squint. These cases usually require frequent and more persistent treatment.

**Partly Curable**—High degrees of errors of refraction, high myopia with retinal degeneration, advance cases of glaucoma, retinitis pigmentosa, macular degeneration, optic atrophy etc.

Never give big promise in such cases. First create movements in the eyeballs and produce relaxation before giving any active exercise.

Do not handle incurable cases. Such cases are mature cataract, absolute glaucoma, absolute optic atrophy, even there is no perception of light. Cases of mature cataract ought to be advised to go to some eye surgeon for operation.

2. Treatment chart is based on two principles—action and relaxation. Arrange the treatment chart in such a way that practice with open eyes is followed by relaxation, along with side exercises.

**Open Eyes**—Active exercises—central fixation on charts. Reading the Snellen eye chart at varying distances, reading of Fundamentals or Fine print in good light and candle light, practice on white lines etc.

Relaxation exercises—as palming, long or short swing, memory swing, imagination of a letter or dot.

Side exercises—game of ball, football swing, writing, sewing, table-tennis, playing cards, walking, musical chairs, reading, puzzles, view cards for art of seeing etc.

3. If the patient takes long treatment in the clinic, arrange the treatment chart in such a way that there is gradual eye

education without any boring effect on the mind of the patient. Change the treatment chart every week or as soon as it is noted that the patient feels strain or no improvement by any particular exercise, or correct the exercise if the patient is not following it properly. Feeling of strain or headache or no improvement is an indication that there is something wrong in the adaptation of the treatment chart or that the patient needs some change in his exercises. Either the patient is doing the exercise in a wrong way or that particular exercise is not meant for him. Do not blame the patient but give constructive suggestions.

4. Make the treatment chart interesting. It is the interest that brings good results.

5. Explain the treatment chart in a simple and practical way and ascertain that the patient understands well and practises correctly.

6. Home Treatment—Write such a treatment chart that the patient may follow it without difficulty. It should be according to his convenience, usually not more than 15 minutes programme at a time. For ordinary cases five minute programme will be enough.

## EYE HYGIENE

According to the accepted ideas of eye hygiene it is important to protect the eyes from a great variety of influences which are often very difficult to avoid, and when people are under these influences, they are thought to be ruining their eyes. Bright lights, artificial lights, dimlights, sudden fluctuations of light, fine print, reading in moving vehicles, reading lying down, etc., have long been considered "bad for the eyes." These ideas are diametrically opposed to the truth. When the eyes are properly used, vision under adverse conditions becomes an actual benefit, because a greater degree of relaxation is required to see under such conditions than under more favourable ones. It is true that the conditions in question may at first cause discomfort, even to persons with normal vision; but a careful study of the facts has demonstrated that only persons with imperfect sight can seriously suffer from them, and if such persons practise central fixation, they quickly become accustomed to them and derive great benefit from them. Hence persons of defective eyesight ought to be educated to use the eyes properly with gentle blinking under adverse conditions for a greater benefit.

Expose the eyes to the sun for a few seconds daily to make the eyes strong.

2. Go to the movies to accustom yourself to sudden fluctuations of light. This will prove very useful.

3. Reading in a bright light and dim light alternately, or going from a dark room to a well lighted room, and *vice versa* are very beneficial.

4. Reading Fine Print daily is extremely beneficial.

5. Reading in moving vehicles helps in improving the sight.

6. Reading in a lying posture is very delightful. Anyone who can read lying down without discomfort is not likely to have any difficulty in reading under ordinary conditions.

The fact is that vision under difficult conditions is a good mental training. The mind may be disturbed at first by the unfavourable environment; but after it has become accustomed to such environments, the mental control and the eyesight are improved.

CHAPTER XIII

## FLOATING SPECKS OR TIMIR

MANY persons suffering from imperfect sight especially myopia complain of specks floating before the eyes; these are called in medical terms "muscae volitantes" or "flying flies." They are usually dark or black but can be of any other colour also, and sometimes they appear like white bubbles. They move somewhat rapidly, usually in curved lines, before the eyes, and always appear to be just beyond the point of fixation of sight. If one tries to look at them directly, they seem to move a little farther away; hence their name is 'flying flies." They may have any shape. They are annoying, and sometimes alarm the patient.

Usually floating specks appear at one time and disappear at another time, but they are often present while one looks towards a uniform white surface. Sometimes they appear when the eyes are closed. Even in extreme cases there are periods, short or long, when they are not seen with the eyes open.

The literature on the subject is full of speculations as to the origin of floating specks. Floating specks are supposed to be due to the presence of moving, floating opacities in the vitreous. They have been attributed to disturbances of the circulation, the digestion and the kidneys and are also supposed to be an evidence of incipient insanity.

**Important Points**—As regards the view that the floating specks are due to the presence of floating vitreous opacities, errors of refraction and physical disturbances, the following points are worth considering:

1. Though floating specks are present usually in high myopia, they are absent in many high myopic cases. On the other hand they may appear before the eyes of persons of fairly good vision or in cases of small errors of refraction. Hence an error of refraction is not the cause.

2. They may be present in some cases suffering from disturbances of circulation, digestion and the kidneys, but they are absent also in most cases suffering from such disturbances even in aggravated state. Further, they are also present in persons who have no such disturbance and are quite healthy. These facts do not tally with the idea that the floating specks are due to disturbances in the system.

3. If the floating specks are due to floating vitreous opacities, then we can safely say that the trouble is an organic one and that the floating specks ought to be seen with the aid of an ophthalmoscope or retinoscope, and that the patient should be able to see them before the eyes when they are open. They should not be seen when the eyes are closed because the retina is sensitive only to light and floating specks can be seen only when the retina is functioning.

On examination with an ophthalmoscope or retinoscope, these floating opacities are not found and the vitreous is usually found to be quite clear. Moores Ball writes in his Modern Ophthalmology. "Muscae volitantes show no opacities to the ophthalmoscope. They are exceedingly annoying, and often remain in spite of the correction of refraction errors and attention to the general health." Moreover, the patient may see them with the eyes closed or in darkness, and may not see them at times when the eyes are open. These facts do not harmonise with the theory that the floating specks are due to the presence of floating vitreous opacities.

4. Suppose there is an opacity in the vitreous of one eye

and the other eye is all right. The vitreous opacity will not be seen as a floating speck because the mind has the faculty of fusing the images of both the eyes. Even if the good eye is covered, the vitreous opacity will not be seen as a speck unless it is quite big, dense and in the centre of vision because the mind has the natural tendency to ignore to see the opacities in the form of speck or specks, just as when there is an opacity on the cornea or on the lens or when the retina has a blind spot, the mind does not perceive a speck before the eye as a result of the opacity or the blind spot. It is why many patients suffering from incipient cataract, keratitis punctata, and central opacity cornea do not complain of speck or specks before the eye though the vision may be defective due to such organic changes. I herewith quote two cases of vitreous opacities, who did not complain of specks before the eyes.

In 1894 A. H. Banson of Dublin, reported the case of a man, aged 62 years, with normal vision, whose right vitreous humour "was studded everywhere with small, smooth, fixed spheres of a light cream colour." (Transactions of the Ophthalmological Society of the United Kingdom, Vol. XIV 1894, p.101)

Regarding the presence of an animal parasite, systicercus, in the vitreous, Moores Ball writes, "In many instances the patient complains only of loss of vision." (Modern Opththalmology)

THEN, WHAT CAN BE THE CAUSE? The truth about the floating specks is that they are the result of a strain of the mind, and when the mind is disturbed for any reason, floating specks are likely to occur. This strain is different from that which causes errors of refraction. In all cases of floating specks it will be found that the central fixation is lost partially or completely. By central fixation I mean that the letter or part of the letter regarded is seen best. For example, there is a small letter

E on the Snellen test card; when the top arm of E is regarded at ten feet or more, it is seen more distinct than the bottom arm of E, and when the bottom arm is regarded, it is seen clearer than the top arm.

As a matter of fact the specks are never seen except when the eyes and mind are under a strain, and they always disappear when the strain is relieved. If one can see a small letter on the Snellen test card at ten feet or more with central fixation and then remember it mentally by central fixation, the specks will immediately disappear or cease to move; but if one tries to remember two or more letters equally well at one time, they will reappear and move. The trouble of floating specks is wholly functional and not an organic one.

Persons who have fairly good vision and see floating specks also suffer from strain. They do not possess good vision all the time. Their central fixation is frequently disturbed by seeing unfamiliar objects, wrong use of the eyes, worries, physical discomforts, lack of good sleep etc. Floating specks may be present before one eye and not before the other, because there are two separate eyes, each functioning separately, one may strain and the other not. All relaxation methods are helpful in relieving the strain.

Patients who usually see floating specks while looking at a white wall or white clouds suffer from strain. Most people who did not see floating specks before, can see floating specks when they look at the sun, or any uniformly bright surface, like a sheet of white paper upon which the sun is shining. This is because most people strain when they look at surfaces of this kind.

The floating specks are present in cases of disturbances of digestion, heart and kidneys because these diseases cause strain on the mind and if the eyes and mind strain in such a way as to cause the presence of floating specks they will appear, otherwise not.

Patients who are bene fited by correction of errors of refraction or by the treatment of the general system are those in whom the strain which makes one see floating specks is somehow relieved along with the correction of errors of refraction or the treatment of the general system.

Why is a patient suffering from floating specks declared to be suffering from vitreous opacities? There are several possibilities:

1. If the opacity is actually present in the vitreous, it will not be seen as a speck unless the opacity is dense and big enough in front of the central vision. The patient in whom there is the presence of the vitreous opacity usually suffers from floating specks as well. It is a mistake to conclude from this that floating specks are due to the vitreous opacity.

2. Opacities in the vitreous may not be found but the doctor explains to the patient that the floating specks are due to the presence of vitreous opacities. It is only for the satisfaction of the patient.

3. Declaration of the presence of vitreous opacity may be due to the fact of the doctor himself suffering from this trouble and hence he sees it in the patient's eye or his mind is already hypnotised by the opinion of great authorities.

TREATMENT: Usually the strain that causes floating specks is easily relieved. Most cases suffering from floating specks have been benefited by the relief of strain with the aid of central fixation exercises and palming. Some cases were cured in a very short time, a day or week, while others took longer time. Seldom there were cases who took very long time, a year or more, for the partial or complete cure.

In the treatment of floating specks it is very important at

first to convince the patient that the trouble of floating specks is merely functional and that there is nothing wrong organically in the eye. The patient is warned not to try with his eyes whether he can see floating specks and is advised to ignore their presence altogether, putting no importance on their presence. Correction of errors of refraction with or without glasses and treatment of physical discomforts help in relieving the strain.

## Stories from the Clinic

1. A patient complained of floating specks before the right eye, especially when he felt tired in the office. He consulted three eminent eye specialists; one of them did not find anything wrong in the eye while the others said that the floating specks were due to the presence of vitreous opacities. He was thoroughly examined and nothing abnormal was found by the examination of urine and blood.

I examined his eyes with the ophthalmoscope and under a strong magnifying glass but I could find no opacities in the vitreous. The patient was suffering from high myopia and using two pairs of glasses, one for distance and the other for reading. I told the patient that there was nothing wrong with his eye. He did not believe me as he was actually seeing floating specks, and because his mind had already been impressed by the opinion of doctors of great reputation. So in order to convince him about my opinion I had to argue with him thus:

"What is the nature of vitreous? Is it not a jelly-like substance?"

"Yes."

"Could a thing, however small, float in a jelly-like substance?"

"No."

"You say floating specks are present especially when you feel tired and only before the right eye. I think they are not present in the mornings when the mind is fresh or when you do not attend office." I added.

"Yes, that is right."

"If the opacities are present in the vitreous, they ought to be present all the time when the eyes are open, and should not disappear when the mind is at rest under certain conditions. Therefore, your trouble is purely functional and can be relieved temporarily in a few minutes by central fixation exercises."

I gave him a book and asked him if he could regard the first word of a sentence more distinctly than the other words. When he regarded the first word with his right eye the word was seen worse than the other words. When the word was regarded with the left eye it was seen as well as other words.

I told him to close his eyes and remember black or white colour any of which he could easily remember. He could remember coaltar colour and felt his eyes and mind relaxed. Then he opened his left eye and looked at the first word for a fraction of a second and noted the word regarded blacker than the others. He then opened the right eye for a fraction of a second but could not note more blackness in the first word. So he closed the eye soon and by frequent repetition he became able to see the word regarded blacker and more distinct than the other words, with each eye separately.

He then practised central fixation on the letters of Snellen test card, and shifted his sight from bottom to top and top to bottom of every letter and noted the part of the letter regarded blacker than the opposite part. In this way he practised even on the smallest letters with each eye.

Then he stood before a window and began to swing a little from side to side gently. He did not care to see anything but merely shifted his sight on the background without any effort to see. He could easily note that the bars of the window appeared to move in a direction opposite to his body movement. At times he closed his eyes and visualised mentally that the window bars were moving in the opposite direction. The patient enjoyed the sun treatment and palming. Gentle blinking was performed when the eyes were open.

By half an hour's practice the floating specks disappeared altogether.

2. Dr. Bates mentions a very interesting case of floating specks in his book. The patient was a physician who had been seen by many nerve and eye specialists before he came to Dr. Bates. He consulted him at last, not because he had any faith in his methods but because it seemed to him that nothing else was left to be done. He had worn glasses prescribed by different doctors without benefit and frequently suffered from headache. Floating specks caused great uneasiness in his surgery work. His treatment proved to be very difficult as his logic was wonderful, apparently unanswerable and yet utterly wrong. His loss of central fixation was of such a high degree that when he looked at a point forty-five degrees to one side of the big C on the Snellen test card he saw the letter just as black as when he directly looked at it. He could not be convinced that this was an abnormal symptom. If he saw the letter, he argued, he must see it as black as it really is, because he was not colour-blind. Finally after some treatment by Dr. Bates, he became able to look away from one of the smaller letters on the Snellen test card and see it worse than when he looked directly at it. When he attained central fixation on the small

letters he experienced a wonderful feeling of rest and floating specks disappeared. Frequently he looked at a blank wall and remembered mentally a small black dot. After some days' practice his sight became normal, and he obtained complete relief from the floating specks and the headache.

3. An old lady patient was suffering from symptoms of glaucoma. Her vision was 6/60 without glasses and 6/6 with glasses of $+3$. She could read bold type about half an inch size at ten inches. She was seeing floating specks which she could multiply and could see them just as clearly with her eyes closed as she could with the eyes open. She was suffering from digestive troubles for a long time. When I asked her if she could see the letter regarded on the Snellen test card more distinct than the other letters of the line of the test card, she said, "I see the other letters, not directly regarded, more distinct than the letter on which I fix my sight." I put this patient under relaxation exercises to improve central fixation. In a week's time floating specks and symptoms of glaucoma completely disappeared. In a month's time the vision was considerably improved.

4. A doctor friend can see consciously at will, any time he desires, floating specks of different colours on looking into the open broad daylight. He notices the strain in the eyes when he is seeing these floating specks. On taking the sight away from the floating specks, paying no attention to them and giving the eyes some rest and relaxation, they are no longer seen.

CHAPTER XIV

# INFLAMMATION OF THE EYE

**Inflamed Eye:** The inflamed eye usually shows the symptoms of redness, watering, sensitiveness to light, pain, dimness in vision etc. According to the parts which are most affected, the inflammation of the eye is called by different names—OPHTHALMIA (general inflammation of the eye-ball), ACUTE CONJUCTIVITIS (inflammation of the conjunctiva), IRITIS (inflammation of the iris), KERATITIS (inflammation of the cornea), SCLERITIS (inflammation of the sclera), CYCLITIS (inflammation of the ciliary body), INFLAMMATORY GLAUCOMA, etc.

**Tension:** The tension of the muscles and nerves of the eye is the most important factor in all the inflammatory conditions. When a person has glaucoma, eye tension can always be demonstrated, because when the eye tension is relieved and corrected, the inflammation of glaucoma subsides. Patients with ophthalmia, iritis, scleritis etc. are suffering from tension. When the tension is relieved, the eye disease disappears.

In some cases, it is more difficult to relieve the tension than in others. No matter whether it is difficult or not, there can be no cure of the eye disease unless the tension is corrected. This tension, besides affecting the eye-ball is also manifest or can be demonstrated in any or all parts of the body. A person who has glaucoma is not only under tension of the eyes, but also under a tension or an unusual contraction of the muscles of the arm, the hand, or all the muscles.

Tension of the internal muscles is always present when a patient has a disease of the chest, and it can be demonstrated that he is also suffering from tension not only of the chest, but also of muscles and nerves in other parts of the body.

There is a tension that contracts the bronchial tubes and interferes with the proper circulation of air into the lungs and out of the lungs. People with pneumonia, tuberculosis of the lungs, or tuberculosis of any part of the body are all suffering from eye tension, and when the eye tension is relieved, the tension in other parts of the body is also relieved. It is an interesting fact that all diseases of the eyes and all diseases of the body are generally associated with eye tension.

A very remarkable case of tension was that of an opera singer who suddenly lost her ability to sing. Specialist of the throat examined her very carefully and they were unanimous in the statement that she had paralysis of the muscles on the left side of her larynx. In connection with this paralysis there was a tumour grown on the left vocal cord. Her symptoms of paralysis were caused by tension, because when the tension was relieved, the paralysis of the vocal cord was also relieved and cured. The tumour which had grown on the left vocal cord disappeared.

There are two things about this case which can be discussed; one is that the paralysis was caused by tension and the other that the tumour of the vocal cord was also caused by tension. When we analyse her case and try to give an explanation of what the tension accomplished, we will probably say a good many things which are not so. It is exceedingly difficult to answer the question, "Why."

We may have cases of eye diseases in which it is difficult to relieve the tension in the eyes but it may be easy to relieve the tension in the muscles of the stomach or in the various groups of muscles in the arm or hand, and when such tension is relieved, then that of the eye muscles is also relieved, and in this way the disease of the eye, no matter what it may be, can always be relieved or cured. This is a very important fact, because when understood and practised, some very severe forms of diseases of the eyes can thus be cured, and in no other way so well.

The question that comes up more prominently than any other is: What can the patient do to bring about relaxation of any group of muscles? A man by the name of F.M. Alexander, of London, has accomplished a great deal in the cure of all kinds of diseases. He says that all diseases of the body are caused by tension. They all can be cured by the relaxation of the tension. He has offered many methods of bringing about relaxation in the most interesting, although seemingly incredible way and the most successful is to bring about relaxation by making the patient say that it is desired.

For example, a patient sitting in a chair or lying down on the floor, whichever is easier, says: "I desire relaxation of the muscles of my neck, so that my head can be lifted forward and upward." This is sometimes repeated a hundred to a thousand times. Mr. Alexander has always succeeded in having the patient bring about relaxation of the muscles of the neck by this method.

Mr. Alexander goes further and brings about relaxation of the muscles of the chest, both outside and inside, by making the patient say: "I wish my shoulder to relax and to move downward and backward. I wish my chest to relax and move backward. I wish my whole body to relax and move backward. I wish my foot to move backward without effort, without strain of any muscles of the body."

It has been a great shock to many orthodox physicians to observe the cures that Alexander has made. Epilepsy, considered by the medical profession to be incurable, has been cured by relaxation, without the use of any other form of treatment. Of course, rheumatism responds perhaps more quickly to relaxation than a great many other diseases, but there are cases of so-called rheumatism affecting the shoulder in which all parts of the joint become immovable.

One patient was afflicted with Parkinson's disease; all the joints of the body became so fastened together, so immovable, that the patient was unable to produce any voluntary movement of the hand or the arm. As time passed, the voluntary and the involuntary muscles gradually became useless from tension. Mr. Alexander had the patient relax those muscles which she could relax most readily. When this was done, the more difficult muscles became relaxed, until finally she was cured completely by the relaxation of tension. Dr. Bates mentions the following interesting case:

"A coal heaver whose face, hands and other parts of the body were covered with black particles of coal, came to the clinic. His right eye was suffering from a hypopion ulcer of the cornea. The case interested me very much and I took him in to see the surgeon in our department, a man who believed very strongly that an abscess in any part of the body is caused by germs, and when there is a collection of pus, it is the physician's duty to drain it and get rid of it. I said to him:

"Would you drain that pus?"

He answered: "Certainly, a man would be crazy not to drain it."

I then said: "Doctor, do you know that some patients in this condition, who have had the pus drained have lost an eye, and oftentimes both eyes, from sympathetic ophthalmia?"

"I don't care, it ought to be drained," he said.

"Just watch me," I said.

Without cleaning the patient's face or eyes, a pressure

bandage was placed over his eye and tied so tightly that his face became much swollen. I told him that in two days, his eye would be cured. The surgeon said:

"Impossible."

I said, "Take a good look at him so that you will recognise him if you ever see him again."

At the end of two days, the man came back, very much annoyed with me. He said that the bandage nearly killed him. "Take it off," I said.

He took it off and the pus had disappeared. The surgeon who saw it said that I had not cured him, that the man did not have an abscess to start with, that he had a perfectly healthy eye, and that anybody who said that the eye was full of pus two days before was wrong.

Strange it may seem, the pressure bandage relieved the tension in the eye to a considerable degree, with a result that the pus in the anterior chamber (hypopion) was entirely absorbed. The eye recovered its health in forty-eight hours and the eyeball became very soft, because the tension was relieved.

It is well to demonstrate the results produced by tension. When the letter "O", for instance, is remembered imperfectly, the white centre becomes a shade of grey and the black part of the letter becomes less black and often covered with a grey cloud. To remember the imperfect letter "O" requires an effort. The effort tires the eyes and mind. The memory of imperfect sight lowers the vision of other letters. When the effort becomes sufficiently great to blur the letter "O" more completely, the tension becomes increased, the eyes feel uncomfortable and may suffer a considerable pain. This pain may be felt in the head, back of the neck, in the arms and in other parts of body.

The memory of perfect sight does not produce fatigue, pain or any other form of discomfort. The memory of perfect sight can be accomplished easily. Any effort, strain or tension spoils it. When the sight is perfect, it is possible for the memory to be perfect, because we can only remember what we have seen; when the memory is perfect, the imagination is perfect, because we can only imagine what we remember. When the imagination is perfect, the sight is perfect, because we can only see perfectly what we imagine perfectly. (B.E.M.)

EFFECTIVE METHODS: Sun treatment, palming, mental pictures and swinging are very helpful methods for relieving the tension. Enema, purgatives, vapour bath, nasal drops, deep breathing and massage are effective methods in the cure of all inflammatory conditions of the eye. Drugs used by mouth or injections should be such that they do not cause any harm to the system.

PAIN: Painful eyes are treated with soothing eye wash and drops. Fomentations or vapour bath to the face and bandaging are frequently done. If there is intolerable pain, mild fomentations are done around the eye and not on the eye; bandage the eye with warm milk cream over the lids. If the pain is accompanied by much redness in the eyes, application of leeches on the temples and vapour bath may also be tried.

THICK DISCHARGE: If the inflammation is accompanied by thick yellowish white discharge (purulent discharge) bandaging is avoided. The eye is frequently washed with lemon juice diluted with water or saline lotion or any other antiseptic lotion. M B 693 or sulphonamide tablets may be given by mouth. Penicillin may be tried. Usually the discharge soon stops, but in some cases vaccine or serum injections are given.

DIET: If there is purulent discharge from the eye, milk, curd, sugar, sour things, potato and meat are contra-indicated.

Green vegetables, fruits, bitters, and bread are to be given. If the inflammation of the eye is not accompanied by purulent discharge, milk, ghee, butter, vegetables, sugar, bread, and rice are useful things; but sour things, oil, meat, brinjal and chillies are contra-indicated.

SWELLING: If there is much swelling of the eyelids, conjunctiva, the following treatment proves very efficacious:

Take some fine ginger powder and dust it on an eye pad. Wash the eye and ask the patient to close the eye; apply a little vaseline on the eyelids and then put the pad dusted with the ginger powder over the closed eyelids. Bandage the eye and let it remain on the eye for an hour at least. The patient will complain of irritation but he should be persuaded to keep it on. This process should be repeated morning and evening. The result in some cases is wonderful. The inflammation soon subsides and the discharge stops.

## After Treatment

When the inflammation subsides the patient is instructed to continue Resolvent 200 or Resolvent 500 or Opacitox Oculose along with sun treatment. If the sight is affected, he is advised to practise central fixation exercises on the Snellen test card and to read fine print daily. He makes it a habit to blink frequently. He practises long swing and palming before and after sleep to prevent eye strain during sleep. Concentration on candle flame while counting 100 respirations is very beneficial.

## Stories From The Clinic

OPHTHALMIA: About two years ago, a patient suffering from ophthalmia with redness in the eyes and wearing dark glasses came to me and narrated the following history:

"Twenty days back I got sudden attack of redness and watering in the eyes and consulted the specialist of the local hospital, who diagnosed trachoma and treated the eyes with caustics. On alternate days the doctor applied coppersulphate on the everted eyelids. Although the treatment was very irritating, I remained under his treatment for 15 days but got no relief. I am getting attacks of headache every morning and the vision is a little hazy. I feel much glare in light and I have to keep up myself in the dark room throughout the day."

I applied Elixir Oculsose in the patient's eyes and placed him on the rocking chair facing the sun. He could not bear the light so I asked him to spread the handkerchief over the face and then rock forward and backward. After five minutes he removed the handkerchief and took sun treatment with the eyes closed for 10 minutes. When he became accustomed to take sun treatment with the eyes closed, I focused the sun rays on his closed eyelids. After sun treatment he washed his eyes in a basin full of cold water by dipping the face frequently in the water.

He then palmed for ten minutes. He practised long swing before and after sleep. Along with the relaxation treatment he was given vapour bath and nasal drops.

On the first day the patient got much relief and on the second day the redness, headache and glare became much less; and in a week's time the patient became all right.

ACUTE GLAUCOMA: A woman suffering from acute glaucoma attended the clinic with her son. Her eyes were congested and she had severe pain in the eyes and violent headache. The lids were a little swollen and the pupils dilated. Her vision was affected.

The first thing we did in her case was to give her a vapour bath and put nasal drops in the nostrils. The nsasal drops were very irritating to the throat and nose. The nose began to run, eyes began to water more, the throat began to caugh. In half an hour about 10 ounces of discharge from the throat and nose was collected in the spitton. After an hours' treatment she felt much relief in her pain and headache.

Locally I gave fomentation and dropped pilocarpine lotion and bandaged the eyes. The attack disappeared on the third day.

To prevent any further attack I advised her to apply Resolvent 200, take sun treatment, do palming and sew in the right way with black thread and white cloth. After two years of the treatment her son reported that she was doing all right.

3. The following case is written by Dr. Bates' assistant.

During the hot summer days while we were still treating patients at the Harlem Hospital Clinic, a little girl named Estelle, about eight years of age, was brought in and placed in the children's ward of the hospital. She met with an accident which destroyed the sight of her left eye. Not being a Clinic case, another doctor took charge of her. One day this doctor came to our room and asked Dr. Bates when he expected to take a vacation. Dr. Bates answered: "I take a vacation every day. Why do you ask?"

The other doctor answered: "I am serious, Dr. Bates. When do you go away for a rest?"

Dr. Bates replied: "When I am treating my patients it rests me, so I don't have to go away. Is there anything I can do for you?"

"Yes," said he. "There is a little girl in the children's ward upstairs and while I am away I would like to have you take care of her case. When I return I shall remove the injured eye, for it is in a bad state and the sight is completely destroyed."

Dr. Bates agreed to take care of the little girl and asked me to help him. We called on Estelle soon after and the nurse in charge of the ward led the way to the tiny cot in far corner of the room. Rows upon rows of cots we passed and on each lay a young child. Some of them were the dearest little pickaninnies you ever saw. A number were crying with pain, while others looked wistful as we passed them by. I could feel their loneliness, away from their mothers, and my heart ached. I glanced at the doctor's face and I could see that he, too, felt sorry for the little ones. Finally the nurse stopped beside Estelle's cot, and the poor child looked very much frightened as the doctor and I came along. We could only see part of her face as she lay there, because the whole left side was covered with a bandage. Before Dr. Bates could say a word to her she began to cry and beg the new doctor not to hurt her like the other doctor. The nurse began to remonstrate with her, but the doctor soon quieted her when he promised in his gentle way that he would not hurt her one single bit. She stopped weeping instantly when the doctor asked her if she would like to see how really funny she looked in a mirror. Was there ever a girl or a woman who did not want to see herself in a mirror? Estelle answered, "But I haven't any mirror."

"Oh!" said the doctor, "Mrs. Lierman always carries one in her purse."

I produced it quickly, before the child lost interest. As she saw the mirror and looked at her bandaged face I noticed that the nurse was bored; all this was a waste of time. She had other duties, undoubtedly, but Dr. Bates believes in taking his time and he surely did on this occasion. The doctor very carefully directed the child to remove the adhesive plaster herself, and in this way the bandage was removed without discomfort or pain. After the doctor had examined the eye, which was almost healed, he turned to the nurse and asked: "Why on this earth is this child kept in bed?" The nurse answered: "Because of the injury to her eye."

"So I see," said the doctor, "but the rest of her body is not sick or injured. Why cannot she get up and walk around here?" The nurse replied: "But I am obeying the doctor's orders."

"All right," said Dr. Bates, "I have charge of her case now, and I think she ought to be out of bed."

Before the nurse could tell Dr. Bates that the child would have to be dressed, he put out his arms towards Estelle and her arms went out towards him with a smile. If our reader has ever visited a patient lying in a hospital bed, why need I explain just what Estelle had on at the time? She didn't care, neither did the doctor. He lifted her gently out of bed, and as she readily gave him her hand both walked slowly down the whole length of the ward. But, coming back, she ran with him. Of course her steps were uncertain, for she had been in bed for two weeks, which made her weak, but she had full confidence in the big doctor who held her hand and who surely would take care that she did not fall. What a funny sight she was! Bare feet, a smile, and practically nothing else. The nurse looked on disdainfully, but I must confess that I giggled. The other children in the ward became interested in the game of the doctor and Estelle. There was a grand exodus of most of the children from their beds, who were anxious to join in the fun. During this time Estelle was not quiet. She was so happy that she screamed with delight, while the other children added their voices to the riot. The nurse had a lively time for fully ten minutes or longer getting things settled again.

To go back to Estelle's trouble. She told us how she had been playing on the sidewalk near her home when she slipped and fell against the kerbstone. A piece of a broken glass bottle lay in her path and it penetrated through her upper closed eyelid and cut the eye so badly that the sight was destroyed completely. Dr. Bates treated the eye later so that it did not have to be removed. Even though she could only see out of one eye, anyone observing her could not have guessed that the sight was destroyed in the left eye.

SWELLING OF EYELIDS AND CONJUNCTIVA: A man got severe inflammation in the left eye. There was much swelling of the eyelids and conjunctiva, and the eye-ball was protruding. He could not close the eyelids. The discharge from the eye was thick and yellowish white. He was treated in the local eye hospital for about ten days but the inflammation did not subside.

The condition of the eye was pitiable. I washed the eye with warm saline and covered it with a wet pad for about 5 minutes. Then I dusted fine ginger powder on a pad and put it on the lids and bandaged the eye. I told him to open the bandage after two hours and then wash the eyes with warm water and apply boric ointment. The same process was repeated in the evening. On the next morning the condition of the eye was quite changed. It was difficult to believe that it was the same inflamed eye. The whole inflammation subsided, the discharge became much less, but the redness in the eye continued. In six days' time the eye gained its normal condition.

PANOPHTHALMITIS: A girl of twelve had acute panophthalmitis due to an injury. The whole eye was under severe inflammation and the pus had formed inside the eye-ball. Profuse thick discharge was running out of the eye. Doctors had advised her father to get her eye-ball removed, as otherwise it might affect the other eye also. Along with the eye wash and eye drops she was given the mixture prepared from the eye discharge. (Mixture:—Take about 4 drops of pus and add to it 4 ounces of distilled water. Dose—I teaspoonfull. On the first day 10 doses, every hour; then on subsequent days, two doses, morning and evening). There was fever on the following night, but the discharge from the eye began to decrease from the second day, and all the inflammation subsided in about 10 days' time. The eye looked all right but she could not regain her vision.

SCLERITIS: A woman had redness somewhat of copper colour in her eyes for six months. There was no swelling of the eyelids, and discharge was absent, but she had uncomfortable feeling in the eyes and glare caused inconvenience in moving about. She was given different treatments for trachoma and conjuctitivitis by several doctors but the redness and other discomforts continued.

I examined her eyes and found that the sclera of both eyes inflamed. I told her husband that she was suffering from chronic scleritis and that she would be all right in about a fortnight. Every morning I applied Elixir Oculose or Resolvent 200 in her eyes just before sun treatment, and gave an eye wash. Swinging proved more helpful than palming. On alternate days vapour bath and nasal drops were given. At bed time she applied sedative antiseptic ointment to check itching and burning sensation. At times she dropped Liq. Adrenalin Chloride well diluted. The eyes were cured in about twenty days' time.

KERATITIS: Inflammation of the eye in most cases is the result of using the eyes wrongly and permitting bad habits to develop. Staring seems to be an innocent habit, but it causes a great deal of trouble. When it is stopped and the eyes are rested by palming, swinging and blinking, the inflammation subsides and sight is benefited.

The Maharajkumar of a Rajaputana State had attacks of

keratitis and ulcer cornea evey now and then. Each attack affected the vision and kept him in bed for about one or two months. He was a patient of many famous eye specialists of Bombay. His body was throughly examined to find out the cause of recurrent attacks of inflammation. His blood was examined several times to see if syphilis was the cause, but each time the result of blood examination was negative. Once he called several eye specialists at a time to examine him thoroughly but they did not give any definite hope that future attacks could be prevented.

I had gone to Ajmer to address a meeting of Princes of the Mayo College. There I gave consultation to the Maharajkumar and found that he was a hypermetropic patient and possessed many pairs of glasses of different prescriptions. The last one was of plus three with plus one cylinder. He could read No. 3 of the Fundamental card without glasses. One could see from the expression of the face that he had the staring habit. Slight redness in the eye was constantly present. He suffered much from glare and had to use dark glasses constantly. I told him that I hoped his eyes would be cured within a few days but he did not believe it.

Treatment of hypermetropia was the right treatment for him. I prescribed Resolvent 500 to be applied in the eyes just before sun treatment, and Ophthalmo to be used after sun treatment. Palming and swinging gave good rest and relaxation. Practice of looking at the white line in between the lines of print greatly helped him to improve the near vision. He learned quickly how to blink and began to do short and gentle blinking. On the very first day of treatment he felt great benefit in his eyes, and after three days' treatment he and others began to say that the improvement in his eyes was wonderful. He could easily read the finest print without the aid of glasses, and could move about freely even in the hot sun without the use of dark glasses. The sclera of the eyes became white and the expression of the face and eyes looked healthy and normal.

He questioned me why I gave preference to fine print and not to large print. I told him that it required more of an effort to see a large letter than a small one; you have to look at a large area of a large letter and usually central fixation is lost in regarding a large area. Loss of central fixation means an effort to see. Fine print is a benefit because it cannot be read while the eyes are under a strain. They have to be relaxed. As soon as you begin to read the fine print while shifting the sight on the white lines, central fixation is improved. He then asked how one could see the letters while moving the sight on the white lines. I said, "While moving the sight on the white lines, the sight shifts to black letters also, but the shiftig is so short and rapid that one does not notice it."

TRACHOMA: Trachoma also is an inflammatory disease. Granules form on the inner surface of the lids. The patient complains of glare, watering, itching and burning sensation, feeling of foreign body in the eye, pain, and defective vision.

Trachoma is supposed to be very common and the use of medicines containing silver and copper is regarded as a specific. It is rather strange that in spite of the numerous hospitals and all possible care the disease is not prevented, and many cases even in the early stage are not at all benefited. Large number of such cases, in spite of continuous treatment, become worse and suffer from other complications even in the hands of experts.

In fact trachoma is not so common as it is supposed to be. Most of the cases, called trachoma patients, suffer from eye strain and that is why they are not benefited by anti-trachoma treatment. Such cases are soon benefited by sun treatment and relaxation methods.

However, trachoma or no trachoma, most patients are remarkably benefited by the use of Elixir oculose or Resolvent or Opacitox Oculose followed by sun treatment, eye wash, palming and reading fine print. In rare cases caustics and even operations are resorted to when the granules are big.

The Commander-in-Chief of Nepal had myopia and frequently used to get redness, watering, foreign-body sensation in the eyes. Several specialists were consulted. All of them diagnosed trachoma, prescribed medicines containing silver and copper, and advised constant use of glasses. Long use of such medicines caused entropion (a condition in which the margin of the lid rolls in due to contraction), and argyrosis (discolouration of the conjunctiva by silver solutions). A Bombay doctor performed entropion operation. His discomforts did not subside and he had to continue anti-trachoma treatment till I treated him when he was fifty-four years old. I told him frankly that he was not suffering from trachoma but from eye strain, and that all anti-trachoma treatment had made his eyes worse; he was simply astonished to hear my words because big doctors treated him for trachoma. I applied Resolvent 500. which was followed by sun treatment, eye wash, palming, swinging, reading fine print and photo print. In a month's time all his complaints disappeared and the vision considerably improved.

A man had big trachoma granules which caused redness in the eyes and other disagreeable symptoms. I performed an operation to press the granules and then occasionally touched the granules with copper sulphate. After some time Opacitox Oculose was prescribed along with sun treatment. The condition of the eyes improved much within a month's time.

SUBJECTIVE CONJUNCTIVITIS: Some people often suffer from subjective conjunctivitis. By subjective conjunctivitis is meant that the conjunctiva is inflamed without the evidence of disease. Many people with subjective conjunctivitis will complain of a foreign body in the eye and yet careful search with the use of good light and a strong magnifying glass will reveal no foreign body present. Some people with the subjective conjunctivitis complain that they have granulated lids and that they suffer from time to time from the presence of little pimples on the inside of the eyelids. The pain that they suffer is out of proportion to the cause that they give to it.

Among the many symptoms of subjective conjunctivitis there may be a flow of tears from very slight irritants. However, the tear ducts, with the aid of which the tears are drained from the eye, are usually open in these cases and they are sufficiently open to receive a soluton of boric acid which may be injected through the tear duct into the nose. This shows that the tear duct is open normally, and therefore can drain the tears from the eyes.

TREATMENT—The patients suffering from subjective conjunctivitis are usually treated by the application of the caustics, drops of silver nitrate, protargol and argyrol etc., and the results are disappointing in many cases; the condition becomes worse in some cases. Liquid Adrenalin is almost a specific remedy for subjective conjunctivitis. It is to be dropped in each eye three times a day. The effect of this medicine is very great if the patient is advised to take sun treatment for a few minutes before dropping the medicine in the eyes. In some cases dry massage of the whole body is very helpful.

FOREGIN BODY IN THE EYE: A woman had pain, watering and redness in her left eye. She was treated in a charitable eye hospital for trachoma for about a fortnight but got no relief. I examined her left eye very carefully and when turned the upper eyelid inside out, I discovered two small eyelashes growing in. This had caused all her suffering, because every time she closed her eye the end of these eyelashes rubbed the cornea of her eye. I promptly removed the two eyelashes with a pair of cilia-forceps and immediately her trouble was over.

Another patient who had pain and redness in the eye was treated medically by other doctors for syphilis. When he did not respond to the treatment the medicine was changed. Then they gave him treatment for rheumatism. The pain still continued, so he attended my clinic. I examined his eye and, found a small foreign body lodged in the cornea. This was removed and, for the first time after weeks, the poor man was relieved entirely of pain. My experience in clinic work makes me believe that in some places charity patients are not always thoroughly examined.

# CHAPTER XV

# DISEASES OF THE OPTIC NERVE
## OPTIC NEURITIS

IT is a common belief that optic neuritis or optic atrophy is mostly due to syphilis or some other infection in the system or teeth. The following facts may be observed regarding optic neuritis cases:

1) Many people suffer from syphilis or some other infection but only a very few out of them suffer also from optic neuritis, and those who suffer from optic neuritis are usually not benefited by anti-syphilitic treatment or anti-toxin treatment or by extraction of teeth.

2) Some cases of optic neuritis do not give any indication, by tests or otherwise, of syphilis or toxin or bad teeth.

3) Some cases of optic neuritis whether they suffer from any infection or not recover partially or completely themselves by rest without any specific treatment.

How can these facts be reconciled with each other if syphilis or some other infection is the cause of optic neuritis?

The following case is a good illustration to explain and reconcile these facts.

S.R. of Delhi, aged 61, was feeling deterioration in the vision of the left eye. For his eye trouble he visited Bombay and consulted two prominent eye-specialists of the place. Both the doctors diagnosed optic neuritis in the left eye and advised the patient to go under different tests. They were of opinion that the condition was a serious one.

The patient's blood, urine and stools were examined in Bombay and Delhi and the sinuses were X-rayed. Nothing abnormal to account for the trouble of optic neuritis could be detected. Wassermann Reaction was found negative. A diagnostic antrum puncture was done and the result was found to be negative. Again new X-rays of the pituitary fossa and the optic foramen were taken, and the Radiologist admitted his inability to pass any judgement regarding the cause of optic neuritis.

I examined the patient with great care. Vision in the left eye was 1/60 faint, which could not improve with glasses. There was total colour blindness. Light-sense had much deteriorated. Biophotometer test revealed that he could see two dots at O degree. The ophthalmoscopy showed signs of optic neuritis. The pupil was normal. Right eye was in normal condition.

His expression of the eye and face indicated that the left eye was under a great strain. My immediate feeling was that the cause of unilateral optic neuritis in this case was eye strain. Moores Ball mentions in 'Modern Ophthalmology' that errors of refraction and eye strain are also the causes of optic neuritis.

But what is eye strain and what are the symptoms when the eye is free from strain and when under strain?

Normally the act of seeing is passive. Things are seen, just as they are felt or tasted or heard, without effort or volition on the part of the subject. When the eye is free from strain, it never tries to see. If for any reason, such as the dimness of the light or the distance of the object it cannot see a particular point, it shifts to another. It never tries to bring out the point by strain at it. If the eye makes an effort or stares at an object, consciously or unconsciously, its normal function is disturbed and imperfect sight is the result. The following experiment is a good illustration:

Fix the sight on any small letter of the Snellen eye chart and then try to see several of them. Soon the letters become blurred, and trying to see them blurs them more.

This shows that imperfect sight is produced by a strain or an effort to see. Let us now consider what are the other symptoms when the eyes are free from strain and when under strain.

1. CENTRAL FIXATION: The retina of the eye has a point of maximum sensitiveness called 'fovea centralis', and the eye sees best through this point. The result is that the letter regarded on the Snellen test card is seen best; other letters in the field of vision appear less distinct. This quality of the eye is called 'central fixation'. When the eye is normal the part seen best is extremely small. When the eye possesses central fixation it not only possesses perfect sight, but is perfectly free from strain and can be used indefinitely without fatigue. Loss of central fixation means strain, and when it is habitual leads to all sorts of abnormal conditions and is, in fact, at the bottom of most eye troubles, functional as well as organic.

2. SHIFTING AND SWINGING: When the normal eye has normal sight it is always shifting from one point to another; it is never stationary. This is true of the eyes closed as well as of the eyes open. It is impossible for the eye to fix on a point longer than a fraction of a second. If it tries to do so, it begins to strain and the vision is lowered. Look at a letter for an appreciable length of time, and note that the letter begins to blur, or even disappear. This shifting of the eye keeps it free from strain.

When the eye shifts slowly or rapidly from side to side, stationary objects appear to move in the direction opposite to the movement of the head and eyes. For example, shift the sight from one side of the Snellen test card to the other, note that the test card and the lines of letters appear to move in the opposite direction. This apparent movement of the object is called swinging. A very simple example of the swing is that experienced in a moving train; the telegraph poles and other objects appear to be moving in the opposite direction.

The shifting of the normal eye is short, gentle and rapid and usually not conspicuous, but by direct examination with the ophthalmoscope it can always be demonstrated. If the eye shifts from one side of a letter to another, the letter appears to move in a pendulum-like motion. The shiftings of an eye with imperfect sight, on the contrary, are slower and jerky and their excursions are wider. The swing of the object is retarded or lost.

Normally the eyeballs move with the movement of the head and any movement of the eyeballs consciously or unconsciously, in the opposite direction of the head causes strain.

3. IMAGINATION: What we see is the mind's interpretation of the retinal images. Take a Snellen test card and hold it at a distance from your eyes at which your sight is fairly good. Look at the white centre of the large letter 'O' and compare the whiteness of the centre of the 'O' with the whiteness of the rest of the card. You may do it readily: but if not, use a screen, that is, a card with a small hole in it. With that card, cover the black part of the letter 'O' and note the white centre of the letter which is exposed by the opening in the screen. Remove the screen and observe that the white centre appears whiter than the margin of the card when the black part of the letter is exposed. When the black part of the letter is covered with a screen the centre of the 'O' is of the same whiteness as the rest of the card. It is therefore possible to demonstrate that the white centre of the 'O' appears whiter than it actually is. That is what Dr. Bates calls imagination. When you see something that is not there, you do not really see it, you only imagine it. The whiter you can imagine the centre of the 'O', the better becomes the vision of the letter 'O' and when

the vision of the letter 'O' improves, the vision of all the letters on the test card improves.

The white centres of the letters on the Snellen test card at 15 or 20 feet are imagined by the normal eye to be whiter than the margin of the card, while the eye with imperfect sight imagines the white centres of the letters to be less white than the margin of the card, or imagines them to be of the same shade. So when the sight is imperfect, not only the eye is at fault but the imagination is also impaired.

So when the eye is free from strain, its action is effortless. It possesses central fixation. The white centre inside the letter appears whiter, and the letter appears to move in the direction contrary to the movement of the eye.

The eye under strain makes an effort to see. Its power of seeing best the letter regarded becomes defective or is lost; the white centres of the letters appear less white; and the apparent movement of the letter is retarded or lost.

If somehow the defective eye can be educated to imitate consciously the qualities of the normal eye, the vision can be benefited. Dr. W. H. Bates M. D. of New York devised some simple eye exercises which readily teach the eye to adopt normal functioning. These exercises have invariably proved very efficacious in the prevention and cure of errors of refraction and in the treatment of the diseases of the inside of the eyeball. It does not take much time to prove their usefulness even in most of those cases in whom syphilis, rheumatism, tuberculosis or any other infection may be regarded as the cause of the disease. Prognosis of the diseases of the inside of the eyeball is usually supposed bad because the patient is not treated simultaneously with the treatment of constitutional diseases, the patient is not given the treatment which can educate the eye to adopt normal functioning. Since eye strain will be found as a common cause in most of the cases, one who can successfully tackle the eye strain will be able to improve the eyesight considerably in most of the cases. The prognosis will be regarded then favourable.

Keeping the fundamentals of the normal eye in view I outlined the treatment for the patient. As the expression of the left eye was that of staring, I asked him to close the eyes and cover them with the palms of his hands avoiding any pressure on the eyeballs, in such a way that no light enters the eyes. This practice is called PALMING. While palming he recalled the images of some black objects as a black shoe, paint, crow, coat, curtain, cap etc. He was able to note that it was all dark before his eyes when they were closed and covered. On the first day he did palming for about 15 minutes and felt as if the heaviness and discomfort were relieved, the eyes were light. After palming for 15 minutes he removed his hands and opened his eyes gently and I taught him how the normal eye blinks. He readily adopted the right blinking. He could easily move his upper eyelids a little to cover the pupil; at times he blinked in a wrong way, that is, he lowered the upper lids so as to touch the lower ones with a jerk. I told him that the habit of blinking was the normal habit and that it was present even in animals and tiny babies, and that blinking was a quick method of resting the eyes. It was a surprise to him to learn that blinking was imperfect, irregular or absent in diseased eyes. It did not take much time to educate him to blink gently and frequently, and in such a way that it does not become conspicuous and that it does not turn into winking.

The next process was to improve the movements or the shifting of the eye. I placed him before a swing stand which is like a window having vertical bars in it. He moved his body and head gently from side to side, moving the sight on the background without making any effort to see things. When he moved to the right, the bars of the swing stand appeared to move in the direction contrary to the movement of his eyes, head and body. The right eye was then covered with an eye shield and the left eye was educated to shift and swing before the swing stand. Unconsciously the eye stared and could not note the swing of the bars. I reminded him frequently not to look at the bars but to move the sight on the background. With the help of frequent palming the eye was tamed to shift without strain.

Then I gave him the Snellen test card and directed him to shift his sight from side to side or up and down of the letters. He could realise the swing in the letters and was able to note that the letter regarded appeared darker than the rest. On the first day he could do central fixation only on two upper lines of the chart, but gradually he could do on all the lines. Whenever he felt any sign of tiredness, he closed the eyes.

From time to time some modifications in the exercises were made and the right eye was kept covered during the time of practice. He was advised to go for driving with the good eye covered and note that the side objects were moving in the opposite direction. From the very first day of the treatment the vision in the left eye began to improve steadily, and in two months' time he became able to read and write. His vision without glasses improved to 6/30, and 6/15 with glasses. He could read Snellen reading type No. 2 with glasses. Colour sense developed fully except for red. Field of vision became normal. Light sense improved considerably.

## Facts Reconciled

The primary cause of optic neuritis is eye strain or mental

strain. If the strain already exists, syphilis or other infections may exaggerate the strain and consequently may cause more damage, but they themselves can hardly cause optic neuritis when there is proper relaxation of the mind and eyes. It is why patients suffering from syphilis or other infections may remain free from optic neuritis, and anti-syphilitic or antitoxin treatment in positive cases may do no good. Cases who recover themselves without any specific treatment or recover by some specific treatment indicate that somehow the strain was relieved from the eyes and mind. Treatment of strain, side by side, with other treatments of any infection will prove really beneficial; but drastic treatment should be avoided as far as possible.

Q.—If the disease is due to strain, then why one eye may be affected and the other remain free, as in the above case?
A.—This is because one has two separate eyes—one may function under strain and the other not.

Q.—Why all persons suffering from mental strain do not suffer from optic neuritis or other eye diseases?
A.—If the mind is under a strain, and yet if the eyes do not make any effort to see, the person will remain free from all such eye troubles; but if the mind is under a strain and the eye also stares, imperfect sight will be the result. The habitual strain may cause diseases of the eye—functional as well as organic.

Q.—Then, why does anti-syphilitic or anti-toxin treatment help considerably in certain cases, if the strain is the main cause?
A.—Syphilis or other infection might be increasing the strain of the mind and eyes, hence anti-syphilitic or anti-toxin treatment helped such cases. Or these cases might be recovering

in the natural course of relaxation and anti-treatment got the credit.

## OPTIC ATROPHY

In optic atrophy a patient usually complains of dimness in the vision and night blindness. His defective vision is not corrected by glasses and the deterioration in his sight gradually goes on increasing. If the defect is not checked, the patient becomes blind. On examination with the ophthalmoscope the optic disc is seen white or grayish. Cases of optic atrophy are commonly supposed to be due to syphilis and anti-syphilitic treatment is administered. Such treatment generally makes the condition worse. Mental and eye strain is the real cause of optic atrophy and relaxation is the right treatment.

### Stories from the Clinic

EARLY OPTIC ATROPHY. A woman aged 35 was wearing glasses for five years. She suffered from headache for about 10 years and had great trouble in reading. A doctor prescribed plus glasses which did not relieve her pain. She consulted many doctors to relieve her pain but everyone prescribed glasses and each prescription differed from the others. The vision was gradually decreasing both for distant and near work. The last doctor diagnosed early stage of optic atrophy with hypermetropia and prescribed some injections, tonics and glasses. All such treatments proved a failure even in the checking of the disease.

Three years ago the patient visited my clinic and I found that she was suffering from hypermetropia and optic atrophy. Hypermetropia is the most frequent cause of discomfort, pain or other diseases of the eye. In her case also hypermetropia was the cause of headache and optic atrophy. The medical men were trying to neutralise the effect of hypermetropia by prescribing glasses but did not try to remove the cause of hypermetropia, that is, a strain at the near point. New methods of treatment in this view are not given any encouragement. A specialist in the old methods would stand up and say: "If I fail no one else can succeed: I know all there is to know about the eye". If one claims to give benefit to a case of optic atrophy, he is regarded as a charlatan.

Treatment of hypermetropia is the right treatment to cure optic atrophy. The cure of hypermetropia is very simple. When one practises in the right way, a cure is always brought about. It takes no more time to practise in the right way than in the wrong way. Hypermetropia is cured by rest, and cannot be benefited by an effort. Practise with fine print is one of the best methods of relieving hypermetropia. The fine print is held first at the distance from the eyes at which the patient sees best and gradually brought closer until the patient can read it at six inches from the eyes. The patient should not look directly at the letters but at the white spaces between the lines and imagine that there is a thin white line beneath each line of letters. Correct practice with fine print daily cures hypermetropia.

In the beginning of the treatment, I prescribed Resolvent 200 which was replaced by Resolvent 500 later on. She liked to take sun-treatment early in the morning as she was afraid of her fair complexion. Palming and swinging helped her much to relieve the headache in a few days. Then I instructed her to practise on the fine print card and photo print. In about two months' time she gained normal vision both for distant and near objects. Signs of optic atrophy disappeared.

If she had any trouble in threading a needle she would hold a needle where there was a background, close her eyes for part of a minute, remembering a small letter "O" while her eyes were closed and this would help her to thread the needle without delay or trouble.

## Complete Optic Atrophy

Nandlal of Cawnpore got injury in his upper teeth at the age of 4 while playing hockey with his brother. Soon profuse bleeding took place and it continued for 10 days. On the 11th day, the doctor gave some injections and the bleeding stopped, but the eyesight was lost. Since then he became blind. He was examined by many doctors who diagnosed optic atrophy in both eyes and treated him for years but he got no improvement in his eyesight. Finally the doctors told him definitely that he would never recover his eyesight and there was no use of spending money.

By the recommendation of one of my patients his brother brought him to my clinic for consultation. His age then was 17. He was weeping and said that he was waiting for death to visit him as soon as possible. I consoled him first and then spent sufficient time in the examination of his eyes. The perception of light was present in the left eye but the right eye had hardly any perception of light. The optic discs in both the eyes were white. I cherished no hope of any benefit, still I wanted to experiment on this case to find out the efficacy of Dr. Bates' methods in such cases. So I told the patient and his brother that there was a little hope of improving the sight and I would like to try the case for a month at least. The patient felt some consolation and it seemed that he had a great confidence in me and had more hopes of his recovery than I had.

I prescribed Opacitox oculose and Retinox oculose to apply in the eyes just before sun treatment three times a day. At times the eyes showed little inflammation so these medicines were stopped for a few days and Resolvent 500 was tried. The rays of the sun were focused with the magnifying glass on his closed eyelids. Palming, he practised many times a day. While sitting on his bed he practised touch swing before and after sleep. In touch swing he kept the eyes closed and put the tip of the thumb on the tip of the forefinger lightly and rubbed the thumb on the finger in one quarter of an inch length. While moving the thumb lightly on the finger he felt as if the thumb was moving on the finger and the finger on the thumb.

He had instructions to keep his eyes closed and to keep himself busy in palming and swinging.In palming there was difficulty of imagining something as he had hardly any memory of the things seen in the past, but he knew music, so I asked him to imagine the rhythm of the music which he could easily do.

His health was very poor and appetite was bad. He frequently complained of heaviness in his head. To improve his general health I prescribed enemas, regulated diet, deep breathing, oil massage for the head and the whole body and Abidol capsules to improve the vitamin deficiency. Once or twice a week he was given vapour bath and nasal drops.

For 15 days I observed no change but afterwards a ray of light penetrated his eyes; it was like a shadow which he could distinguish vaguely when somebody appeared before him. Gradually the shadow took a shape of reality until he was able to distinguish colours of objects. He began to walk without the help of an attendant. One day he was walking with some patients. A crow was sitting at some distance; one of the patients asked Nandlal if he could see anything in his front. Nandlal said that some black thing was there. Later on he was able to distinguish some letters on the Snellen test card at six inches. The improvement was quite slow in his case but he and I were quite satisfied with it. The patient left the hospital after two month's treatment.

## Shock and Optic Atrophy

The following case is from Dr. Bates' clinic and the history is written by Emily C. Lierman.

On July 16, 1923, there came to our office a man suffering with blindness caused by a sudden shock. As I stood before him and asked him what his trouble was, his eyes looked up towards the ceiling and immediately I noticed that he could not see me. He had been sent to us in the hope that Dr. Bates would be able to restore his sight. Previous to his visit on that day I received a telephone message from a woman employed by the Compensation Bureau of the City of New York. She told me that he was blind and it was the opinion of the eye specialists consulted that there was no hope of his sight ever being restored. Dr. Bates examined his eyes with the ophthalmoscope and found that he had atrophy of the optic nerve and that he was under a terrible tension.

With each eye separately he could see the 200 line letter of the test card at one foot temporarily. He could only do this in flashes, because he stared continuously, which blinded him. The variable swing improved his vision to 6/200 and his field was also improved by the swing. He came daily to the office for treatment, and on the 21st. of July he read 9/20 after he had palmed his eyes for a long time. Sun-gazing outdoors improved his vision also. His general depression became less and he informed me that he was feeling much better after each visit. For a long time he did not have very much to say but after he had become better acquainted with us all, he began to talk about his case. He had been working in the moving picture studios for quite a few years and apparently he felt no discomfort in his eyes. This is the story he told me:

"I was standing on the top rung of a ladder readjusting electrical parts used in the studios for taking moving pictures. At the time there was just an ordinary light such as is used in most offices. Without my knowing it, a strong Kleig light was suddenly turned on and I received a sudden shock which caused blindness instantly. I was taken care of, as are other employees in the studio, and then was taken home. Since then I have not been able to work. It seemed as though my troubles were multiplied when my little baby boy fell sick and died. I had no money with which to bury him until my wife's parents came to our aid. Christmas came very shortly, with no hope of Christmas cheer for my other child, a little girl just three years old. We were in debt, but I had planned, when I was able to work again, to pay back the money which was used to bury my baby. My wife tried to console me and make me feel that things were not quite so bad, but I saw no hope ahead of me on account of my blindness."

We felt all the more here at the office that our patient should have all the treatment that could be given him in order to restore his sight, if possible, and we worked diligently all through the Fall and Winter with steady results.

During the month of May we had many rainy days with very little sun. This patient had demonstrated to us that the sun is very necessary for the eyes. During all these months of almost daily treatment he had no such poor vision as he had in the last few weeks. His vision was lowered to 10/50 and he became very much discouraged. After the sun had shone for a day he came to the office feeling light-hearted and happy. He

was given the sun treatment and immediately his vision improved to normal, reading 10/10 at times. The doctor questioned
his ability to dodge automobiles at the crossings here in our big
city. His answer was that he could get along very well on bright
days when the sun was shining, but he still feared the traffic
on rainy days. While this conversation was going on the patient
was looking very intently at the Doctor's face as he stood about
three feet away. He did not move an eyelash, but just stared
all the while he talked. He had forgotten the very thing that
helped him, blinking. All of a sudden he exclaimed: "Doctor,
now as I look at you, you haven't any head."

"No," the doctor replied: "seems to me the other day
somebody told me I did have a head. But you never can tell;
some people don't always tell the truth."

Immediately the patient apologised and hastened to say:
"Oh, but doctor, when I come close enough to you I can see
that you have a head."

Dr. Bates has always advocated the movies. Whenever a
patient stares he advises him to go to the movies. Dr. Bates
enjoys them himself and goes as often as he is able to.

We owe a great deal to the moving picture artists, for a great
part of their work is done under unfavourable conditions.
The Kleig light, while it is powerful, is not injurious to the
eyes of the actors and actresses when their eyes are properly
used. Most of them work under a terrible tension, with the
feeling that their eyes will be injured by the strong glare. A
great many eye specialists no doubt have treated injury to the
eyes apparently caused by the Kleig light. The light would be
harmless if those who work in the studios could keep their
minds relaxed and if they could also understand and use our
method—resting the eyes all day long.

Dr. Bates discovered many years ago the benefit of strong

light on the eyes and I have seen many patients cured by the sun treatment alone. Some of these cases were seriously affected because of their inability to stand even the rays of the sun. It is curious but true that this patient has been benefited mostly by a magnifying glass which focused the light on the white part of each eye as he looked down while the upper lid was raised. In the beginning of his treatment the mere mention of light would make him frown and shrink with fear. Now he enjoys sitting in the sun all day long and realizes that it gives him the greatest benefit. He is steadily improving. While he is not entirely cured, he reads the bottom line of the test card occasionally at ten feet.

He has great hopes of being cured and is so grateful of what has been done for his eyes that he insists upon my writing to two of our most popular actresses of the screen who are interested in his case. We are striving to cure him so that we can send a note of thanks to those who are interested in him and to try and encourage others, who might be troubled by the Kleig light, to come to us to be benefited as he was.

# Chapter XVI

## EYE EDUCATION

### See The Natural way

*Preservation of good eyesight is almost impossible without proper eye education and mental relaxation. The quieter the mind, the better is the eyesight preserved.*

It is a fact that glasses help many to relieve their discomforts of their head and eyes and enable people to see well at a distance or near, and their use in many cases is imperative. But this is also true that glasses do not check further deterioration and the number of glasses goes on increasing. Often glasses become an added torture to increase the pain and suffering and loss of eyesight. The fast deterioration in eyesight and the development of some serious complications are not prevented by the use of glasses, injections and pills. Therefore, the number of blind people amongst the educated class is fast increasing in spite of all possible medical aid.

The orthodox belief is that for cases of defective eyesight as myopia and hypermetropia and astigmatism, there is not only no cure, but practically no preventive also. Any rational mind will think such a claim as dogmatic, an imperfection in the ophthalmic science. When the sight begins to deteriorate, there must be some cause for it, and the cause is always an effort to see or strain. The eye being a sense organ is closely associated with the mind in its functioning, and like other sense organs makes no effort to see in its normal course. The normal eye when it makes an effort to see at a distance, its distant vision becomes defective and myopia is produced. When the normal eye makes an effort to see at a near point, its near vision becomes defective and hypermetropia is produced. Glasses neutralize the effect of such conditions but do not relieve the cause of the trouble. So, in many cases, the cause continues increasing by the use of glasses and the sight goes on deteriorating.

It is a well known fact that vision is a process of mental interpretation. The picture which the mind sees is not the impression on the retina, but a mental interpretation of it. For example, to the good eye the white centre of letter O seems to be whiter than the margin of the page, this is because the mind interprets the retinal image in this way. Therefore, our vision mostly depends on our mind's imagination. When the imagination is perfect, sight is perfect. But if the imagination is imperfect, sight also is recorded imperfect.

The old writers on ophthalmology did not consider that the mental strain could play an important part in the formation of errors of refraction, hence they isolated the eye while determining the cause and treatment of visual defects and retinal disorders. To rectify the effect of errors of refraction they prescribed glasses. But very little has ever been claimed about their usefulness except that these contrivances neutralize the effects of the various conditions for which they are prescribed, as a crutch enables a lame man to walk. This incurability of errors of refraction is based on the theory that the eye changes its focus for vision at different distances by altering the curvature of the lens.

It struck to Dr. W. H. Bates M.D., an American Scientist, that further experiments and observations were necessary to determine the facts about accommodation and errors of refraction. His experiments are a proof that the lens is not a factor in accommodation. The eye adjusts its focus for different distances just like a camera, by a change in the length of the organ, and this alteration is brought about by the action of external eye muscles called oblique muscles. Dr.Bates has made many remarkable discoveries regarding the refraction of the eye but the most remarkable discovery of Dr. Bates is: **Fine print is a benefit to the eyes while large print is a menace**. The reason is that while reading fine print one sees a tiny area at a time, while in reading large print one has to see a large area at a time and the eye feels strain in such an attempt.

Dr. Bates' discoveries are a boon to humanity. Thousands of cases, so-called incurable, have been benefited by his simple methods of treatment. For example, a woman who had developed total night blindness was completely cured in about a month's time. And a boy who had become semiblind, gained normal vision in a couple of weeks. A German lady who had developed squint by the wrong use of the eyes was cured in about two weeks time. Cases of incipient cataract, glaucoma, retinal disorders, floating specks, amblyopia, etc., have derived great benefit by the system of eye education.

All along it has been my experience that mental relaxation is the key to success in life, in education and treatment. Under the present conditions of life, man's mind is under a severe strain, hence preservation of good eyesight has become almost impossible without eye education. One may have good eyesight today but will not be able to preserve it after some time. If children and adults are taught about the proper use of the eyes, most of the visual defects will fade away in due course of time and man will enjoy perfect eyesight. Though glasses are also necessary in some cases, yet unless the prescription of glasses is supplemented by eye education deterioration in eyesight and blindness cannot be prevented.

*Blind Notions:* Reading fine print is commonly supposed to be harmful to the eyes, and reading print of any kind in dim light and close to the eyes is regarded as a dangerous practice. Due to such a belief a student suffered a lot. He had pain in the eyes and pain in the head, he was in a state of agony and lost his peace of the mind and his health was affected. When he began to read fine print in candle light and good light alternately at a close distance, surprisingly all his pain in the eyes was chased away in three days and was relieved from headache. Details of these blind notions may be studied from the book *'Yoga of Perfect Sight'*.

## Variations in Eyesight

Refraction of the eye is never permanent. The normal eye does not maintain perfect eyesight all the time. If the eye is defective, its error of refraction does not continue the same; there are moments when even bad eyesight cases see better or worse. Therefore myopia and hypermetropia are not constant conditions to the same degree.

When the normal eye makes an effort to see distant objects, its distant vision becomes defective; and when it strains to see near objects, its near vision becomes defective. Similarly when the defective eyesight cases are able to lessen the effort to see consciously or unconsciously, their sight is found to be better. Even during sleep the refractive condition of the eye is usually found to be worse; this is why people in the morning wake up with eyes more tired than at other times.

When the eye regards an unfamiliar object an error of refraction is always produced. Hence fatigue is caused by viewing pictures or other objects in a museum. Seeing a map at a distance produces myopia. Children learning to read, write, draw or sew often suffer from defective vision because of the unfamiliarity of the lines or objects with which they are working.

All persons see imperfectly when they hear an unexpected loud noise. Familiar sounds do not lower the vision.

Under mental strain or physical discomforts as pain, cough, fever, depression, anger, fear, etc., errors of refraction are always produced.

A sudden exposure to strong light or rapid changes of light are likely to produce imperfect sight.

Changes in the refraction is responsible for many accidents. When people are struck down in the street by automobiles or cars, it is often due to the fact they were suffering from temporary loss of sight.

The error of refraction is lessened by seeing familiar objects, hearing familiar sounds, rest and relaxation and other favourable conditions but this variation is diminished by wearing spectacles because the eye tries to maintain the same error of refraction as that of the lens.

## Concentration and Relaxation

What is concentration? The dictionary says concentration is an effort to keep the mind fixed on a point or to fix the gaze on one point or on one letter or an object. Such a thing is impossible and always causes great strain and those who practise it suffer from imperfect sight and mental strain, and then lose the power of concentration. Their memory, imagination and sight are affected. For example, concentrate your mind and eyes on a part of big letter of the Snellen Test Card at ten feet, the gaze is fixed at one point. Within a few minutes you will observe that the vision begins to blur, the strain in the eyes and mind becomes evident.

But if by concentration you mean, doing or seeing one thing better than anything else, and shifting the sight from one part to another, then you may speak of concentration, it is then central fixation. For example, look at a small letter on the Snellen Test Card and shift the sight from side to side, observe that the letter appears to make short movements from side to side and the part regarded appears best. This kind of concentration is immensely beneficial to the mind and eyes.

Recent psychology gives a new interpretation to concentration. Attention underlies concentration. The state of attention which seems to be continuous is in reality intermittent; the object of attention is merely a centre, the point to which attention returns again and again. All parts of the object, and then the reflections inspired by these various parts hold our interest by turns. Even when the attention is fixed on the most trifling material object, it works in just the same fashion. This is entirely according to central fixation as described by Dr. Bates.

There are two aspects of concentration—voluntary and involuntary. Voluntary concentration is an effort and cannot be maintained without fatigue; our thought holds the object in focus. Whereas in involuntary concentration there is no effort, the object holds our thought without our volition as in contemplation and meditation or in central fixation.

Involuntary concentration and relaxation are the same thing. Relaxation of the passive kind usually ends in sleep or sleepiness, as experienced by many patients in palming. Relaxation combined with action as usually one experiences in swinging, central fixation and white line of fine print is also free from effort and strain when done properly.

Another thing about relaxation: obstacles to relaxation may prove sources of relaxation. An instance of which is found in the noise that is keeping us awake when wishing to go to sleep. If we sufficiently relax, if we accept the disturbance and sleep in spite of it, not only is the obstacle overcome, but because overcome, it in turn becomes rather pleasantly associated with going to sleep. When again we desire to sleep, we find the noise soothing rather than annoying, and really a source of relaxation instead of an obstacle to it.

## How To Concentrate

To remember the letter O of fine print continuously and without effort proceed as follows:

Imagine a little black spot on the right-hand side of the O blacker than the rest of the letter; then imagine a similar spot on the left-hand side. Shift the attention from the right-hand spot to the left, and observe that every time you think of the left spot the O appears to move to the right, and every time you think of the right one it appears to move to the left. This motion, when the shifting is done properly, is very short, less than the width of the letter. Latter you may become able to imagine the O without conscious shifting and swinging, but whenever the attention is directed to the matter these things will be noticed.

Now do the same thing with a letter on the test card. If the shifting is normal, it will be noted that the letter can be regarded indefinitely, and that it appears to have a slight motion

To demonstrate that the attempt to concentrate spoils the memory, or imagination, and the vision:

Try to think continuously of a spot on one part of an imagined letter. The spot and the whole letter will soon disappear. Or try to imagine the whole letter, equally black and distinct at one time; this will be found to be even more difficult.

Do the same with a letter on the test card. The results will be the same.

CHAPTER XVII

# PRESCRIPTION OF GLASSES

PRESCRIPTION of glasses is usually done by the help of a trial case. The trial case is a box containing plus + and minus— lenses, spherical and cylinderical, beginning from 0.25 to 14 or more. Besides trial lenses there is a trial frame, a black disc to cover the eye and a piece of velvet to clean the lenses. The power of the lens is written on the lens. Cylinderical lenses have a mark to indicate the axis.

## How to Know the Kind of Lens ?

1. Move a spherical lens before the eye and look at an object. The object will appear to move. If the object appears to move in the opposite direction, the lens is convex or plus. If the object appears to move in the same direction the lens is concave or minus.

2. When a cylinder is moved in the direction of its axis, no movement of the object is visible, but in the other position the object appears to move in the same direction or in the opposite direction.

3. The power of the lens is determined by neutralization. Lenses of the opposite kind are taken from the trial case and placed in front of that to tested, and moved before the eye. The neutralizing lens is the one which stops all apparent movement of the object.

## Some Important Rules for the Prescription of Glasses

1. The patient reads the Snellen test card from 10 or 20 ft.

and if he can read ten feet line from 10 ft., or twenty feet line from 20 ft., his sight is recorded normal or almost normal, no glasses are necessary for distance. If the patient can read the fine print at 9 to 14 inches, his vision for reading is normal and no glasses are necessary to see near objects.

2. If the patient is unable to read the normal line on the Snellen test card but can read fine print all right, he is probably myopic. So try minus lenses to bring the sight to normal. The lowest power which gives normal vision, is the number for that eye. Each eye to be examined separately.

3. If the patient cannot see fine print at any distance, he is probably hypermetropic or presbyopic. Try convex or plus lenses. The patient will need that lens which gives clear vision to read fine print.

4. A myopic patient usually does not need glasses for near work because his eyesight is very good for reading. However, if he is using glasses for reading and complains of headache and strain and discomfort, he needs either no glasses or less power for reading.

5. If the patient is using convex lens for distance, he will require higher power for reading, especially when he is at the age of forty. And as the age advances, the power of the reading lens is also increased.

6. If the sight is normal for distance then at the age of forty one usually needs+ 1.0; at the age of fifty,+2.0; at the age of sixty,+3.0. If the patient is hypermetropic or myopic, his distant number is added to these figures.

7. In presbyopic patients tell the patient to hold the book at his convenient distance to which he is accustomed. Some hold the book at 12 inches, others at 16 inches. Accordingly find out the number which gives good vision and proves comfortable.

8. If one eye is hypermetropic or normal, and the other is myopic, patient does not need glasses because one eye is working all right for distance and the other eye for near.

9. If there is a great difference in the number of two eyes, try to give number to both the eyes in such a way that the difference does not exceed more than two diopters, otherwise mind will find it difficult to fuse the images of the two eyes and in due course of time memory of the patient will be affected due to mental strain.

10. Some patients resent to glasses and get headache even if the number is quite high. In such cases the use of glasses should be limited to necessity only.

11. In many cases after the age of fifty or sixty near vision begins to improve and the patient can either discard the reading glasses or requires the lower power.

12. If the patient has astigmatism and requires cylinder, then the same axis is maintained for distance and near, only the power of the spherical lens is increased or decreased.

13. Bifocals are prescribed for persons who frequently look at a distance or near as judges, teachers, advocates, etc. The upper lens is meant for distance while the lower lens is meant for reading.

14. If one eye is good and the other operated for cataract, give no glass for the operated eye, otherwise double vision will appear and that will be very annoying to the patient.

15. If the patient complains of discomforts with the spectacles:
   a. The glasses may not be correct.
   b. The eyes resent to glasses.
   c. The cause may be psychological.
   d. Frame may not be fitting and the lenses may not be clear.
   e. The patient continues the habit of straining.

202 SECRETS OF INDIAN MEDICINE

16. If the patient is using plus lenses for distance and often gets headache, it is better to discard the glasses for distance for some time and then if necessary give less power.

17. If myopia is not high and the number is constant then it is harmless myopia. It will greatly help in old age. The patient will not need glasses for reading and he will be free from many a trouble of old age.

18. Myopic patients should be advised not to use glasses in reading. Reading fine print daily will greatly help them to maintain good eyesight.

# CHAPTER XVIII

# TREATMENT OF MYOPIA

MYOPIA or shortsightedness is an error of refraction. The sight is usually very good at about ten inches or nearer while very dim or blurred for objects at ten feet or farther. The eyeball is elongated and the eye cannot focus for distant objects. By putting concave lens before the eye the distant objects appear clear.

The cause of myopia is strain or an effort to see at distant objects. Rest of the eyes and mind is the cure for myopia. How can people with myopia be conscious of a strain? This is an important question. When methods are practised in a wrong way or practised unsuccessfully, a strain or an effort to see better can usually be felt, demonstrated, or realized. Look at the top letter of the Snellen test card at ten feet distance. Try to see the top and bottom of the letter at a time and equally well. Observe that the smaller letters become dim. Now close the eyes and touch the closed eyelids with the tips of the fingers lightly and observe that there is increased hardness of the eyeball.

Quite frequently it is difficult for people with imperfect sight to believe that perfect sight requires no effort and that any effort to improve the sight is wrong. It has been so habitual to strain, and the habit of straining to improve the sight, the memory, or the imagination, has been practised so long that it requires sufficient time and patience to stop.

It is not true that myopia is caused by too much use of the eyes at a near point. On the contrary, near use of the eyes in a poor light lessens myopia. The treatment of myopia which I have found best is as follows: the vision of each eye is tested and the patient is then directed to sit with the eyes closed and covered with the palms of each hand in such a way as to avoid pressure on the eyeballs. At the end of half an hour or longer, the patient is directed to stand with the feet about one foot apart and sway from side to side as he reads the Snellen test card at five feet or ten feet.

Some cases obtain a decided improvement in their vision by the memory of a known letter. The patient is told to look directly at one letter of the Snellen test card for five seconds while blinking frequently, the letter has been committed to memory. When the eyes are closed, the memory of a known letter is usually better than when the eyes are open. By alternately regarding a letter, closing the eyes and remembering it better than when the eyes are open, the vision of this letter will improve in most cases. The more perfectly a letter is remembered or imagined, the better becomes the sight. When a letter is remembered or imagined as well with the eyes open as with the eyes closed, a maximum amount of improvement in the vision is obtained.

Some cases are benefited by teaching the patients how to make their sight worse by staring, straining, or making an effort to see. When the cause of the imperfect sight of myopia becomes known, the vision often improves to a considerable degree. When myopic patients learn by actual demonstration the cause of their trouble, it makes it possible for them to improve their sight.

Myopic persons who desire a cure should discard the use of glasses. Just putting glasses on for an emergency for a few minutes may bring on a relapse and what was gained may be lost. In some cases the improvement is considerable in a short time but then does not go further, in such cases a lower number is prescribed and the patient is asked to use the glasses when necessary to see the distant objects but not for reading. Side by side the patient devotes a few minutes to maintain his improvement.

Some myopic patients are unable to stand bright light. Many doctors prescribe dark glasses for the benefit of such cases. In my experience, wearing of dark glasses is an injury rather than a benefit. One of the best methods to relieve the intolerance of light is to encourage the patient to face the sun with eyes closed for a few minutes daily.

Shifting the gaze from one point to another or side to side of a letter on the Snellen test card may be done in such a way as to rest the eyes by lessening or preventing the strain. Staring or shifting with an effort always produces myopia. Moving the head and eyes from side to side produces an apparent movement of stationary letters or other objects. A complete rest of the eyes with improved vision may be obtained in this way.

Reading in candle light or in dim light for long hours lessens the degree of myopia, so such a practice is greatly advisable. It is a wrong belief that reading in dim light causes myopia.

One of the best methods of obtaining relaxation is to move the ball of the thumb lightly against the ball of the forefinger in a circular direction in which the circle has a diameter of less than one-quarter of an inch. Just moving the thumb in this direction does not always succeed unless one can count one, three, five, or more odd numbers, when the motion is downwards, and an even number when the thumb moves upwards. It is not necessary for the patient to watch the movement of of the thumb in order to keep up the practice. Dizziness or headache which is caused by strain of the eyes and mind is relieved most successfully by this practice. One can practise while sitting or walking or going on a staircase or while seeing the cinema.

Recently we had a number of myopic cases ranging from - 1.0 to - 19. We found that almost all were greatly benefited by eye education and mental relaxation. Some gained normal vision within a week or so, in some the power of glasses was considerably reduced. One case of high myopia of —12 who could read only the top letter of the Snellen test card from ten feet, greatly surprised us when the patient could easily read the last but one line of the chart and felt no difficulty in moving about and in reading his books from 9 or 10 inches. In one case myopia was followed by the detachment of retina in the left eye and the eye was almost blind. After a month's practice the vision of this blind eye considerably improved and the patient began to read and write.

## Case Report

It is believable that a person while at death bed and given up as a hopeless case by eminent physicians, can regain his life and vitality by prayers, or some simple treatment or by the touch of a saint. But it is unbelievable that a high myopic patient can have considerable improvement in his vision without glasses by rest and relaxation. Many high myopic patients have shown considerable improvement by the system of eye education. There were some failures also, but that was due to improper practice of eye education. However, one case has greatly surprised every one present when she read last but one line without glasses after ten days treatment.

Raji, a girl of 12 years, wearing thick glasses attended the School for Perfect Eyesight with her uncle who is an engineer at A.I.R. Pondicherry. At the age of 5, Raji showed occasional squint in her eyes. Later on, she suffered from irritation and watering and redness in the eyes and had frequent headache. Due to these discomforts she could not read her lessons in the school. She was taken to Madras, there the Ophthalmic Surgeon prescribed glasses:

R.E. - 6.5 Dsph - 1.25 Dcyl. axis 180

L.E. - 10.0 Dsph - 1.25 Dcyl. axis 180

As her discomforts of the eyes did not subside in spite of the constant use of glasses, another eye specialist was consulted a year later and he prescribed another pair of glasses:

R.E. - 8.5 Dsph - 2.5 Dcyl axis 180

L.E. - 10.0 Dsph - 2.5 Dcyl axis 180

The girl was still suffering from the same troubles, so she was taken to JIPMER, there the Ophthalmic Surgeon prescribed another pair of glasses:

R.E. —9.0 Dsph —2.0 Dcyl axis 180

L.E. —12.5 Dsph —2.0 Dcyl axis 180

The parents got disgusted by the prescription of glasses as Raji continued to suffer and this suffering was increasing. When her vision was tested on the Snellen test card from 10 feet, it was recorded 10/200 without glasses and 10/50 with glasses. Her look was a presentation of some great strain, she stared to see objects and did not blink, as if it was a fixed gaze. The Ophthalmoscope did not reveal any organic change. Her colour perception was found quite normal.

It is a fact when the normal eye makes an effort to see distant objects and tries to see a large area at a time equally well, it becomes defective and the retinoscope reveals myopic refraction. When the normal eye strains to see at near in dim light, it adopts hypermetropic refraction. It means the refraction of the eye changes according to the strain and relaxation. So Raji was taught how to use the eyes without strain. By different methods of eye education she learnt how to keep the lids in the right position and blink gently and frequently. To relieve the sensitiveness to light and to relieve the tension of the eyes she faced the morning sun daily for a few minutes and then after a saline eye wash sat comfortably and practised palming.

By palming I mean to close the eyes and cover them with the palms of the hands in such a way that no light enters the eyes and there is no pressure on the eyes. When a person with normal sight practises palming, he experiences all perfect dark before the eyes while palming but myopic patients usually fail to observe perfect darkness and this is a symptom of imperfect relaxation. However, when Raji practised palming, she observed that it was all perfect dark before her eyes when they were closed and covered. She felt that palming was very soothing to her head and eyes, even to her whole body. After ten minutes palming she ran around a chair, while bouncing a ball and after a few rounds she read the Snellen eye chart with gentle blinking from 3 ft. As her improvement in vision was quite fast, the chart was removed from 3 ft. to 5 ft. and then to 10 ft. At times she went to the dark room to read small print in candle light, this was a great help to improve her eyesight. We have found that reading fine print in good light and candle light alternately proves extremely beneficial and gives instantaneous relief in many cases who suffer from eye strain and headache.

After ten days treatment Raji gave a great surprise to every body present at the time of eye examination. She could read the last but one line of the eye chart from ten feet and her vision was recorded 10/20, that is almost normal. How it has happened, a surprise but a fact also. She is relieved from all the discomforts and now she is very cheerful. The expression of her face is quite changed.

Another case, a boy named Akshaya, son of Dr. Indra Bhargava, was wearing glasses of —2.5 in the right eye, and —2.0 in the left eye. In about two weeks treatment by eye education his number of glasses came down to —1.75 in the right eye and —1.25 in the left eye. The boy was advised to use the glasses for distance and to avoid their use in reading.

Some myopic patients do not show good improvement in spite of their interest in the treatment, and it is difficult to explain why some respond very well while others do not. Anyway all are benefited more or less, hence prevention is possible in almost all cases. This is the superiority of eye education and mental relaxation to all other methods—glasses, injections and pills. Now we have some definite methods for the prevention and cure of defective vision even in cases of retinal disorders and in this respect science has much advanced but human mind as yet is very conservative. Our Ophthalmologists are not ready to study or experiment the subject and if you approach to the Government to varify the usefulness of the system of eye education so as to give benefit at large, there is no response. Thus the humanity suffers and the number of blind people amongst the educated class is fast increasing. But a time will come when this dull consciousness of man will change and we will adopt such simple and sure methods for the benefit of the humanity. To the persons of good will, study of the books CARE OF EYES and YOGA OF PERFECT SIGHT to know something more in detail is advisable.

A patient relates his experience in this letter:

"Almost every eye specialist of the world believes that for the refractive errors there is not only no cure, practically no preventive also. From such a belief any rational mind will conclude that Ophthalmic science is yet in a very imperfect stage.

"I was having myopia from my childhood and was wearing glasses of —4 at the age of 5. We consulted many eye specialists who were supposed to be topping their profession. They could not do anything except correcting the defective eyesight with higher power of lenses. I felt that task of wearing glasses very palling, but I did not have any other alternate remedy. At the age of 20 the power of the lens was enormously increased to —12. Moreover my right eye was blind for about 15 years. It was troublesome to go out in the dark without a guide.

"Fortune focussed its rays on me one day. Our family doctor informed my parents that in Pondicherry Ashram there is one Doctor Agarwal curing cases like that of mine. But I was the one who denied to understand all this and refused to go to Pondicherry for my treatment. Finally my parents persuaded my mind.

"On the 13th March 1971 I came with my father to the holy land of Pondicherry and met Dr. Agarwal at the School for Perfect Eyesight. Doctor Agarwal removed my wrong conception about the new system of treatment and asked me to take off glasses which is very necessary to bring any good improvement. He was injecting enthusiasm everyday by telling me that I was improving quite fast.

"The treatment schedule includes sun treatment, palming, long swing, reading in candle light, moving around the round table and special bandage which they call Tarpana treatment. The effect of this Tarpana was observed really wonderful. My eyesight began to improve quite fast. Even the right eye which was absolutely blind began to perceive light and the left eye was found greatly improved.

"Now I am completing the course of treatment of two months. Everybody is surprised to see my improvement. I no more use glasses. My power has come to -5 but the use of glasses gives some discomfort so I don't like to use them. There is no difficulty in moving about or in reading without glasses. The right eye which was blind at one time, can read the letters on the chart."

## NYSTAGMUS

When the eyes move conspicuously from side to side, regularly or continuously, the condition is called nystagmus. So seldom are eye diseases with nystagmus cured that many doctors believe that most cases with nystagmus are incurable. I have found that most of these so-called incurable cases can be greatly benefited or cured.

We have observed that many eyes with imperfect sight do not have nystagmus but acquire it by a stare or effort to see. In many cases nystagmus has been relieved by relaxation with the aid of palming and swinging and reading of fine print. When a patient of nystagmus is able to read fine print or photographic type reduction, nystagmus is cured. The patient is told to glance at the white lines in between the lines of print with gentle blinking.

A girl patient had developed nystagmus and her vision both for distance and near was very poor. Glasses did not improve her sight. In her case, palming, drawing, running in a circle while bouncing a ball and reading smaller print several times a day, proved most beneficial, both for the nystagmus and vision. Her sight to see distant objects considerably improved and she became able to read fine print and photographic type reduction.

Recently we had a very interesting case of nystagmus. A teacher, albino from birth, with white skin and red pupils due to lack of pigmentation, was on a visit to Sri Aurobindo Ashram and while passing through the Romain Rolland Street of

Pondicherry entered the School for Perfect Eyesight. This patient knew me through my articles published in Mother India, a monthly journal of the Ashram.

Since childhood this patient named by Upadhya had very bad eyesight due to presence of nystagmus and the eye experts of his area were of opinion that nothing could be done to improve the defective vision and nystagmus. The objects and letters and words of the book appeared flickering and this unsteadiness in the vision was a great handicap. However, just to help, the reading glasses of $+7$ were prescribed; this helped his reading a little but the strain in the eyes and mind grew more and more. Frequent changes in the number of glasses did not help him either.

When this patient rested his eyes for a long time after facing the sun with eyes closed, it was observed that nystagmus lessened and the vision improved but when he made an effort to see or stared at an object, nystagmus increased and the vision lowered. By repetition he was convinced that his eyes could be benefited by rest and relaxation of his eyes. When he stood before a window he could observe easily that the short or long swing helped him to relax his eyes. Concentration on a candle flame while counting twentyfive respirations and reading of Fundamental chart alternately proved very successful in his case. The congenital nystagmus almost stopped and there was no flickering of objects or words. He could read the smaller letters of a book. Yet he needed an aid of glasses, so a glass of $+3.0$ was prescribed for reading and this was a good help to him.

## TREATMENT IN THE CLINIC

In the treatment of eye diseases the methods which are at hand with the orthodox ophthalmic practitioners for the visual defects are of little value. They neither prevent nor cure the trouble. When a patient complains of defective eyesight, usually glasses are given. Some of the cases develop fast deterioration in eyesight and are given up as hopeless cases. When there are symptoms of cataract or glaucoma in the eye, patients are advised operation. Cataract patients, of course, need operation when the cataract is in mature stage, but some cataract patients have to wait for many many years while glaucoma cases are seldom benefited by operation. Diseases of the retina are rarely benefited by the usual treatment. At first most of the time and money are wasted in finding out the cause of the diseases by various laboratory tests and yet often without any result. Most of the patients are declared as incurable sooner or later. Patients who have no organic trouble but suffer from loss of sight are treated in various ineffective ways. In short, the present system of treating diseases of the eye and its discomforts are very unsatisfactory.

A student had the habit of reading under high power of electric light upto the middle of the night. Gradually his sight began to fail and he felt difficulty in seeing when he came from light to darkness. He started seeing floating specks before the eyes. He was taken to several eye specialists and was thoroughly examined by various tests but there was nothing wrong in the system. Finally the doctors of Orissa declared that his retina was under degeneration and the chances were of becoming blind in future. Each time atropine lotion was used to examine his eyes, the condition became worse. All this was a great shock to the boy as well as to the parents. For several months the boy was under treatment at the Cuttack Medical College and many injections and tablets were tried but with·out any good result. When the parents got disgusted with this kind of experimental treatment and prayed, someone informed them about the School for Perfect Eyesight at Sri Aurobindo Ashram, Pondicherry. And one day I found the father and the son sitting in the reception room and waiting for my consultation.

For the examination of eyes we rarely use atropine or any other medicine for dilatation of the pupil. Nowadays the electrical instruments for the examination of the eyes are so good that the eyes can very well be examined without any dilatation of the pupil. Dilatation of the pupil causes strain and sometimes very severe strain. A patient developed blindness after the use of atropine. So this student was examined without any atropine drops. His eyesight was recorded, his field of vision was taken, his colour sense was observed and his eyes were thoroughly examined in the dark room. It is true that his retina was showing some signs of unhealthy retina.

The father felt very happy when I said that the boy would be all right in a few months and there was nothing to worry. When asked about the cause of the trouble, I said that there was a great strain on his eyes due to reading under high power electric light, the glare reflected from the paper was the source of this strain. Other factors as constipation, poor action of the liver and poor health had helped the trouble to increase.

The boy had developed the habit of staring, he did not blink at all while reading or seeing things at a distance. So the first thing in the treatment was to teach him to blink gently and frequently and we adopted various methods in this direction. Often he played with a ball and moved the ball from hand to hand while shifting the sight with the ball with blinking. While walking he blinked at each step. When he began to blink properly, it was amazing how the floating specks got disappeared and the strain was relieved to a great extent. Frequently he practised palming for ten or fifteen minutes at a time, and this had a good effect to relax his eyes, mind and the nerves of the whole body. Reading of fine print in good light and candle light alternately helped him greatly to read ordinary book print without any strain. At the end of eye exercises such as swinging and central fixation his eyes were bandaged for about half an hour with some medicine pads. Once a week he was advised to clear the bowels by an enema. His diet was regulated with more fruits and greens. The result was that his health considerably improved and the eyes became all right.

Almost every patient faces the sun with eyes closed or with gentle and frequent blinking after the application of Resolvent 200. In some cases the rays of the sun are condensed with a magnifying glass on the closed eyelids or on the white part of the eye with frequent movements from side to side to avoid the heat of the rays. This procedure is greatly helpful in clearing the vision and improving the health of the eye. After the sun treatment eyes are washed with Ophthalmo eye lotion and the patients are advised to practise palming to relax the mind and the eyes. After palming each one follows different exercises according to the prescription. It is frequently noted within a few days how wonderfully the so-called incurable cases begin to improve their eyesight. When necessary glasses are also prescribed or an operation is advised.

We have evolved a system of practical working in the School for Perfect Eyesight based on the synthesis of all the systems of medicine. We believe that all the methods of treatment as glasses, medicines, operation, eye education and methods of relaxation, have their value, but one has to discriminate what is necessary in a particular case. However, eye education and relaxation treatment is prescribed for everyone at least to prevent further deterioration. The efficacy of eye education and relaxation is so great that sometimes one can successfully treat cases of serious eye troubles even without a diagnosis. The reason is that whenever a patient complains of pain, headache or loss of vision, it is an indication of eye strain and mental strain; and the treatment which will relieve the strain will be beneficial to the eyes. An elderly patient gave a history of constant pain in the eyes and gradual loss of sight and inability to sleep at night. Every doctor who examined her admitted that he did not know what was wrong. Blindness was expected by some doctors in the course of a few years. I told this lady patient that I too did not know what was wrong organically in her eyes but I believed that she could be all right by eye education without entering into the details of diagnosis. She followed the treatment quite devotedly and became all right within a short time. The details of eye education and relaxation may be studied from Mind and Vision and Yoga of Perfect Sight.

To some cases of defective vision we advise to take a course of Tarpana Treatment. The effect of Tarpana treatment is to relieve the tension and to make the vision clearer. The process of **Tarpana Treatment** is as follows:

1. Melt the Tarpana medicine in hot water by placing the bottle of Tarpana in it.

2. Make a thick paste of wheat flour by adding water to it. Put the paste on the cotton pads and then put a thin layer of cloth over the paste. When the pads are ready, put a thin layer of Tarpana medicine with a rod over these pads.

3. Fill the eye cup with warm water to which about half the dropper of Tarpana (about 15 or 20 drops of Tarpana) is added. Mix well. Then wash each eye with fresh preparation for two minutes.

4. After eye wash with Tarpana wipe the eyes with cotton or a napkin. Then put the wheat flour pads over the eyes and

bandage them. Bandage is to remain for two hours or till morning. If there is any painful discomfort, the bandage is to be removed.

5. When the bandage is opened wash the eyes with warm water to which about 20 to 30 drops of Ophthalmo is added. Wash each eye for two minutes. Then wipe the eyes and apply Elixir Oculose.

6. Precautions—Light diet. Avoid to see bright objects, lights, fire, sky. No reading, no strain to see things. Better remain in the dark and keep the eyes closed or go to sleep.

7. Tarpana bandage is to be repeated for 3 days or as directed by the doctor. Best time for Tarpana is evening time and when it is neither too hot nor too cold. One can take Tarpana treatment at bed time also.

8. Symptoms of successful Tarpana—Good sleep, no headache, comfortable feeling in the eyes, vision better, light eyes, no itching sensation, no glare.

## DETACHMENT OF RETINA

Detachment of retina is a frequent occurance in high myopic patients; the disease makes the eye blind and the patient is found under a terrible strain of the mind and eyes. Adoption of right blinking, frequent palming and reading of fine print is the sure preventive for the detachment of retina.

What is the treatment for the detachment of retina? Operation is usually a failure. Cases of detachment of retina spoiled by operation can hardly be benefited; treatment by relaxation methods is the right thing. A girl patient from Calcutta, named Upama Pan, suffering from high myopia got detachment of retina in her left eye about two years back. Doctors of Calcutta gave up the case as a hopeless one. This patient got her vision back in about one and a half months time by the system of eye education and relaxation. The followig letter about a case of detachment of retina treated earlier is very interesting and informative:

"I began to use glasses of -1.0 since the tender age of 13 and have been wearing them regularly, but to my utter misfortune, instead of improving or at any rate, preserving my sight status quo they went on rather rendering it worse and worse day by day with the result that those that I am using at present are of - 13.0. One day, all of a sudden, I felt an absolute absence of visual power in my right eye and my consequent consternation can better be imagined than described. I hurried to Patna to receive a medical aid and I was admitted to a paying cabin of the Patna General Hospital under the advice and care of the Eye Specialist in-charge and to augment my anxiety in course of my treatment for ten days there was no improvement whatsoever. I had however, to leave the Hospital in sheer despair and disappointment. Subsequently I consulted the retired eye specialist of the P.G.Hospital and placed myself under his treatment. Both the doctors were unanimous in their diagnosis that the case was one of *detachment of retina* with haemorrhage and prescribed one and the same medicines. They wanted to give sub-conjunctival injections in my right eye. Their treatments for about a month with all their fame and experience did me little good and they ever lulled me to patience by suggesting that I could hope for progress only little by little with the result that the protracted hope instead of bring ing on any substantial relief ended in bitter disappointment.

"Fortunately I consulted Dr. R.S. Agarwal and placed myself under his treatment. He directed me to undergo some very simple ocular exercises and the marvellous result was that hardly a month and a half were over when the visual power of my right eye was restored and I can read now even the fine print. It is interesting to note that the faculty of sight has grown still sharper than before. The myopia in both the eyes has wonderfully considerably decreased. The letter that I could hardly see at the distance of 2 feet can now be seen distinctly at 20 feet or more." B. L. RASTOGI

Operation may be necessary in certain cases to replace the retina but unless the patient is taught how to relax the mind and eyes, he may have no improvement or may lose it soon. After all why was there detachment of retina? It was due to severe strain on the eye. So it is necessary to teach the patient blinking, palming, swinging etc. The difficulty is that the doctor recons those cases in which the success is gained and the failures are not numbered.

## MACULAR DEGENERATION

There is a tiny area in the centre of the retina with which we see best where we are looking. Suppose there are two letters R and B, placed at one inch apart. When R is regarded, R appears better than B, and when B is seen, B appears blacker than R. This tiny area of acute vision is called central spot or macula. When the macular area shows signs of degeneration as seen by the instrument Ophthalmoscope, the condition is called degeneration of macula or macular degeneration. The vision is greatly affected and the patient's mind and eyes are found under a great strain. The affected eye is unable to read and write and often sees floating specks before the eyes. Sometimes the straight things appear curved and the colours appear differently. There is no treatment for such a trouble with the orthodox ophthalmic practitioners. But by proper eye education and mental relaxation the vision can be restored partially or completely.

The most common symptom in macular degeneration is that the faculty of the eye to see best where it is looking, is lost, in other words central fixation becomes very very defective. When tested on the Snellen test card, the letter regarded appears less distinct than the others placed by the side and the white space of the letter appears less white. The look of the patient indicates an expression of severe strain and the eyes appear, as if fixed in the bony socket.

A young man one day observed that his right eye did not see anything. The doctors of Calcutta whom he consulted diagnosed 'Macular degeneration' and told the patient that his right eye was lost and there was no treatment for such a trouble. Somehow this patient came to know about me and wanted to follow the treatment. He had a good understanding. When I explained some of the relaxation eye exercises as frequent palming, long swing, blinking etc., he could do them to my satisfaction. The result was that after a few weeks the vision was restored. When this patient met me again after some years I found that the improvement was very well maintained though the macular area was still visible in a degenerative condition. The eyesight of the affected eye was found better than the left eye which was apparently normal.

This patient was re-examined by the doctors in Calcutta and they were surprised to see that the affected eye was giving better vision than the unaffected eye though the macular area was still diseased.

# CHAPTER XIX

## HEALTH AND ILL-HEALTH

(This chapter is written in the form of questions and answers. The questions were put to me by a person.)

*Q: How to fight out cold?*
A: Cold is a form of illness caused by some disequillibrium and disharmony in the body. It usually manifests as running of the nose, heaviness, headache and fever. Ordinarily cold is due to accumulation of toxic matter and the Nature tries to expel it through the nose or burn it through fever, especially in persons who are more sensitive and mentally developed. When the digestion is weak, bowels constipated and gases formed, the toxin accumulates in the body cells and brain cells. Usually eating fat, sugar and cereals in excess, lack of exercise and mental disturbance cause indigestion and constipation. Such cases are cured by regulating diet, a fast now and then, exercise and relaxation. In two or three days time the running of the nose stops, the toxin is eliminated and one feels a happy feeling and energy in the body; but if this toxin is not allowed to flow out by taking some medicines and injections, then the toxin will first create some functional disturbance and then may affect the organs. A girl aged nine, sensitive and intelligent, fond of sweets, frequently suffered from the running of the nose. Parents being afraid went to a doctor who treated the girl patient by some injections, probably penicillin. Running of the nose completely stopped and after a short lapse of time her activity became dull and the memory became weak. Another case, a man while suffering from acute attack of cold continued his

usual diet containing sufficient clarified butter, milk, sweets etc. The result was that the discharge became thick and could not flow out easily and this caused discomfort in breathing and the trouble became chronic. He then consulted a physician of an old school who asked this patient to take guavas with lemon and chillies and as much as he could and in diet fried horse grams and barley flour bread were recommended. The result was that the accumulated mucous passed out with stools and the gram-barley diet helped in drying the watery portion of the toxin. The patient became all right within a few days. There was a Naturopath in Delhi who could cure an attack of cold within a few hours by giving a strong enema which brought out one or two pounds of mucous with stools. The toxin which would have taken several days to flow out in a natural course could be expelled so quickly. How the enema acts? Enema fluid in the colon draws morbid matter lodged in the entire body from the foot to the head, just as the sun in the sky sucks up the moisture from the earth or a cloth sucks up the pigment from the water dyed with colour. In this respect Charaka mentions various prescriptions used for an enema.

When there is no accumulation of toxic matter due to indigestion and constipation, even then one may suffer from cold due to weak vitality, exposure to sudden change of weather, fear or an attack of hostile atmosphere. In such cases tea, warm decoctions, tonics, rest, joyful atmosphere are very helpful. In the case of a spiritual person who leads spiritual life in the right sense, the matter is somewhat different. His outer trouble is connected with the inner condition. The light of the Spirit tries to lighten the entire human being, the tissues and the body cells which ordinarily begin to decay from the middle age. In this process of creating more energy and light in the body cells the toxin is being eliminated through the running of the nose to rejuvenate and transform the body cells. This suffering may be short or long at intervals but finally the spiritual force can create so much vitality and energy in the body that the person will be free from any kind of attack of cold. Any kind of treatment in such cases to check the flow of the toxic matter worsens the condition. A person sensitive by nature, frequently suffering from cold, leading a spiritual life, consulted a Homeopath who prescribed a medicine of high potency. Of course, the running of the nose stopped within a few hours but discomfort and cold in the body increased. This discomfort was relieved when again the nose was allowed to run through some artificial means.

*Q: How to find out one's own right quantity of food?*

A: Food is meant to feed the physical, the body, which has an instinct and tells you what and how much food is to be taken. This instinct is quite prominent in animals but in man due to developed intellect and perverted desire this instinct is dulled, yet one can understand by experience what is needed for health. The difficulty is that one might be knowing well what is good for health, yet out of sheer greed one overloads the belly. It is why indigestion and constipation with their allied complications and diseases are present in persons who are mentally developed. Usually after 35 or 40 years of age a change takes place in the whole human system and it is at this middle part of life that most people suffer mentally and physically. People try to continue the same quantity of food which their body could easily bear formerly. Towards the middle age to cut the quota of fat, sugar and cereals and meat is very helpful. To replace the quantity of heavy food one should add fruits, green vegetables, milk and other light articles. In the young age cells of the body grow and naturally such foods containing more proteins, fats and carbohydrates are needed for the growth, but in the middle age the growth is stunned and decay starts. So to maintain the balance of health light diet is very beneficial.

*Q: How to discriminate between Sattwic, Rajasic and Tamasic food?*

A: This is difficult as one does not usually understand what is Sattwa, Rajas or Tamas. However, I shall explain in an interesting way through poetry.

### Choice of Food

Enjoy food with mind at ease,
Eat what thy system needs
Without haste in a clean place
And take *rasa* without greed.

Quantity sufficient in right measure,
Neither more nor less, without eager.
Masticate well what you eat.
Eating too much gives you dis-ease.
Find the balance the body needs,
Eating too little makes you weak.

But what shalt thou eat,
Sattwic, Rajasic or Tamasic diet?
The Gita details in this way,
Select the food, thy nature likes to take.
A Yogi's diet is Sattwic food.

The body decides what is to choose.
To nourish the mental, vital, physical force,
To increase the pleasure and happy dose,
For inner and outer strength giving,
Select the diet soft, firm and satisfying.

## Sattwic Food

Milk, curd, bread soft and cheese,
Butter, cream, honey and sweets,
Cake, biscuit, burfi, Rasogolla,
Sandesh, Rasomalai, Sohanhalwa,
Fresh fruits, banana, apple and grapes,
Almond, raisin, figs and dates,
Salad, porridge and chop potato,
Juice fruits, milk cow, and soup tomato,
Vegetables warm, pulse and rice,
Varieties are these of Sattwic diet.
Fresh, flavoured menu attracts the taste
But eating too much is a mistake.
A piece of lemon, bitter gourd and cauliflower
Keep you happy, lighten the heart and liver.
A cup of light tea, coffee or Ovaltine
Relish the taste, digestion increase.

## Rajasic Food

Foods violently sour, hot and pungent
Are liked by Rajasic temperament.
Articles rough, strong and burning
Invite ailments, ill-health giving.
They heat the blood and spoil the health.

Avoid such articles in inflammations and eyes red.

Look to the shop of Punjabwala,
Sells the meat, fish, Pakori mirchawala.
Smell strong invites Rajasic people,
Calls you to sit at the dining table.
Varieties many to create heat in the body,
Tell your desire and pay a rupee.
Mango pickles, vinegar chatni burn the tongue,
Vegetables full of chillies, garlic and onion.
Dosha he gives with a cup of Rasam,
Offers a bag of 'Chana Jor Garam'.
Asks you to taste a dish of roasted hen
And take a dose of whisky or wine.
Tea strong, coffee strong or ice cream
Namkin, sweets, egg-froth or what you need.

### Tamasic Food

Food cold, impure, stale, of rotten nature
Gives to Tamasic temperament a perverse pleasure,
Virtues gone, taste gone, flavour gone;
By Sattwic man such articles ever thrown.
Harmful to health, dulls the mind;
Given such food to animal kind.

See the old man and his dirty shop
Sell the rotten meat and stale chops.
Foul smell keeps you away
But attracts the Tamasic man to foodstale.
Vegetables and Namkin of several days,
Flies on fish, sweets and cakes.

Fruits rotten, insects inside and outside,
Milk sour, curd sour, bread dry.

*Q: What is the effect of Asanas and Pranayam?*

A: Various postures of Asanas cure the restlessness of the body and give to it health, force and suppleness. Pranayam, the control of the breath, increases the vitality, gives robust health and prolonged youth.

*Q: Is it possible for any individual to resist decay and illness?*

A: Yes, one can be entirely free from illness and decay through Yogic force and can lead a happy and healthy life as many Yogis did in the past but the absolute immunity can happen only in a person in whom the Supramental Force has descended and supramental change has taken place in the body.

Life is in the process of evolution. From matter it has evolved as plant; then mind element entered in life and animal has evolved. Man is a thinking animal, the highest evolution so far has taken place. Now the element of Supermind will manifest. There is a vast difference between the consciousness of an animal and man. Man is a constant puzzle to an animal. The same vast difference will happen between man and super-man. It is very difficult for the mind to understand what this superman would be. The Supramental force manifesting in a person will transform the human into superman. He would have the human shape yet quite different inside. He will be constantly in contact with the Divine and his body will contain enormous energy and force which will make his body immune to illness and decay. His force and light will radiate in the atmosphere and he will be the saviour of the humanity. In this respect Sri Aurobindo has written in detail in his book Life Divine, Synthesis of Yoga, Bulletin of Physical Education Vol. I.

*Q: What are the values of Vata, Pitta and Kapha to a modern mind?*

A: Vata, Pitta and Kapha are symbolic terms which the Rishis discovered through the inner knowledge to express the art and science of medicine in a simple way. A true grasp of the subject makes the art of medicine easy and simple and initiates the intelligence to adopt the right course of treatment otherwise the intellect wanders like a thirsty deer in a desert. Now a days a specialist can treat cases only of those diseases in which he specialises, his knowledge becomes limited, but by proper understanding of Vata, Pitta and Kapha one can be an all round good physician and also a specialist.

These terms can be widely used at each step of medicine and I give here a few illustrations on the next page. The discrimination is according to the context. Homeopathy selects other synonyms for Vata, Pitta and Kapha—Psora, Syphilis and Gonorrhoea.

# SOME ILLUSTRATIONS OF VATA, PITTA, KAPHA

## SOME ILLUSTRATIONS OF

| | CONTEXT | PARTICULARS |
|---|---|---|
| 1 | Gross body | Head, chest-abdomen, arms-legs |
| 2 | Systems | Nervous, respiratory, Digestive & Circulatory, Muscular |
| 3 | Function | Mind, vital, physical |
| 4 | Gunas | Sattwic, Rajasic, Tamasic |
| 5 | Cell | Nucleus, protoplasm, body of the cell |
| 6 | Humors | Air, gastric juice, saliva |
| 7 | Excretions | Exhaled air, urine, perspiration, faeces |
| 8 | Expulsion of dosha | Wind, watery or yellow discharge, mucous |
| 9. | Feeling of dosha | Pain or dryness, heat, cold |
| 10 | Classification | Painful or paralytic, inflammatory, non-inflammatory diseases |
| 11 | Causes | Lack of relaxation, low vitality, accumulation of toxic matter |
| 12 | Treatment | Relaxation, stimulation, elimination |
| 13 | Nature | Air, sun, earth or moon |
| 14 | Shape | Gases, liquids, solids |
| 15 | Profession | Judge, police, scavenger |

# VATA, PITTA, KAPHA

| VATA | PITTA | KAPHA |
|---|---|---|
| Head | Chest—abdomen | Arms-legs |
| Nervous and respiratory | Digestive & circulatory | Muscular |
| Mind | Vital | Physical |
| Sattwic | Rajasic | Tamasic |
| Nucleus | Protoplasm | Body of the cell |
| Air | Gastric juice | Saliva |
| Exhaled air | Urine & perspiration | faeces |
| Wind | Watery or yellow discharge | Mucous |
| Pain or dryness | heat | cold |
| Painful or paralytic diseases | Inflammatory diseases | Non-inflammatory diseases |
| Lack of relaxation | Low vitality | Accumulation of toxic matter |
| Relaxation | Stimulation | Elimination |
| Air | Sun | Earth or moon |
| Gases | Liquids | Solids |
| Judge | Police | Scavenger |

T 16

CHAPTER XX

# PERFECTION OF THE BODY

## Health and Vitality

OUR health and vitality depends on how we eat and drink, think and work and regulate our life. It is a general belief that the more we eat the stronger we become, but the truth is that the more we eat, the weaker we become. Over eating often makes a person fat and this corpulence appears in many ways. If you desire to thicken the mental activity of an intellectual, feed him well. Often we plan our eating and drinking more carefully than other more important things. Excessive nutrition does not increase vitality. What nutrition is to the human body, fuel is to an engine. Over fueling cannot increase the horse-power of an engine but can destroy the machine.

Just as a machine needs coal, various kinds of oils and water, so also man needs different kinds of nutrition—carbohydrates, proteins, fats and also water to make the human machinery work properly. Disease and mortality are often due to over-eating. Therefore to restore health the first thing is to regulate our nutrition.

Our food must be in proportion to the requirements of our body and nature of work. A mental worker needs less food but of better quality than a labourer. What is good for one may be positively harmful to another, hence we should choose our diet according to our experience suitable to our condition and constitution. This is also true, what is excess in one case may be insufficient in another. However, nature's instinct is a good guide about the quantity and quality of food.

When a person feels weak and even exhausted in spite of taking his usual meals, the cause is probably in the stomach. The remedy in such cases is to adjust the diet first and give sufficient rest to the stomach in between the meals. By regulating diet and by rest the false weakness disappears, the patient feels energetic and finds no difficulty in doing his usual work. Therefore one should eat at fixed hours, reasonably, calmly and quietly. Do not eat too much, eat just what is necessary. Give up all desire and attraction, all vital movements. When you eat only because the body needs food, then the body will tell you in a precise and exact manner when it has just the amount necessary. It is only when you have notions in your mind or desires in your vital for a particular item, that you eat in multiples of the quantity needed and oppress your body and make it lose its natural perception.

To maintain good health man's mind and body need some physical exercise of some kind or some physical work. This helps his digestion and relaxation. To restore vitality proper sleep is also essential.

Digestive troubles and nervous disturbances usually go together. The doctor should deal not only with the body of his patient but also with his mind, because the mind works upon the body. But the state of the mind depends upon man's consciousness. A good doctor will consider all these points while giving the treatment to his patient. He will adopt simple and harmless methods of treatment which will bring quick recovery to his patients. His very presence will radiate peace and confidence in his patients.

## Mental Attitude

Man is a thinking being. To think is to reason, and to reason means to distinguish between right and wrong. The source of evil and noble thinking is within us. Noble thoughts come from the higher nature or the powers of the soul; evil thoughts come from the lower nature. It is by developing the higher nature that the lower nature can change. All human faculties become weaker with age but by the power of the spirit they can become stronger and stronger and enlightened. The secret of joyous life consists in removing our mind from selfishness and should think more for the good of others. Peace of the mind preserves vitality, while mental agitations rob us of vitality. Anger, fear and over-anxiety greatly lower the vitality and the consciousness. An impulsive person who cannot control himself has a disordered life. To develop the peace of mind two things are necessary.

1. Adjust the diet properly, do some exercise or physical work or Asanas and sleep well.

2. Devote some time in silence and develop the peace and force of the soul.

Concentration upon oneself means unhappiness. Concentration on the soul or the Divine alone brings joy and delight in life. All our sufferings disappear by the realisation of the Divine. To love truly the Divine we must rise above desire and attachments. Only he who loves can recognise love. Those who are incapable of giving themselves in a sincere love, will never recognise love anywhere.

## Human Complexities

There are infinite number of cells in the human body.

These cells are spread over the whole body and do different work in different parts. Those in the digestive system select from our food exactly those substances which they need. These requirements are known as salts, vitamins, hormones, enzymes, etc. But when the cells are damaged by over-eating or wrong eating or under-eating, the system fails to get the proper requirements and the human machinery gets disturbed, symptoms of disease begin to appear. The role of medical science is to restore the activity of the cells on the lines of nature and not by drastic measures. Peace and stillness are great remedies for the treatment of diseases, especially in diabetes and high blood pressure. When we can bring peace into our cells we are cured. It is in peace that the body can reject illness as energetically as in the mind we reject falsehood.

## Sex-Energy

The sex-energy is a great power, it is a support of the body and its vitality. It has two components, one meant for procreation and the other for feeding the general energies of the body, mind and vital—also the spiritual energies of the body. The old Yogis call these two components *retas* and *ojas*.

The sex-energy utilised by Nature for the purpose of reproduction is in its real nature a fundamental energy of life. This energy can be controlled and diverted from the sex-purpose and used for aesthetic and artistic or other creation. When entirely controlled, it turns into a force of spiritual energy. This was well known in ancient India and called by the name of *brahmacharya*. Sex-energy misused turns to disorder and disintegration of the life-energy and its powers.

In the supramental body the sex-energy will be fully controlled and diverted upwards for the transformation into spiritual force. It will be secreted enormously and sublimated immediately into spiritual energy, radiating its light and force into the cells of the body, thus keeping the body hale and hearty, free from decay and death. The whole sex-machinery is renewed by the supramental power to function indefinitely.

## Superman

There is an ascending evolution in nature which goes from stone to the plant, from the plant to the animal, from the animal to man. Because man is, for the moment, the last rung at the summit of the ascending evolution, he considers himself as the final stage in this ascension and believes there can be nothing on earth superior to him. This is his mistake to think like that. In his physical nature he is yet almost an animal, a thinking and speaking animal, but still an animal in his material habits and instincts. Desires, attachments, doubt, selfishness, fear and anger are often expressed in his life, and he is not free from pain and suffering, decay and old age. Undoubtedly nature cannot be satisfied with such an imperfect result; her attempt is to evolve superman, a being who will appear as a man in its external form, and yet quite changed inside. He will be conscious of the Divine in him and will be the embodiment of love and power, doing great works for the upliftment of humanity in joy and Ananda. He will be quite healthy physically and the capacities of his nature will be greatly heightened. The cells of the body will be full of light and force, free from disease and decay. He will be immune to any infection and to the ignorant attacks of the world. He will constantly draw energy from the universe to keep himself fit for the work. He will bring down the divine Powers and Delight from the

Heaven to the earth to establish peace, love and delight in the world. Then the divine life will be established and man will work in truth and harmony.

## Psychology

To understand man and his nature and his mental development is called psychology.

Man is not only a superficial mind but also a more enlightened mind. The superficial mind of man is something like that of an animal which is limited by the conditions of the physical parts of his being and cannot break the limits of his covering and become something greater than the present self and cannot become a more free and noble being. But man by a deeper mental power can break the limits of his vital and physical being, he can develop in him a still greater energy called supramental power which can break all the restrictions; with that power man can achieve the divine nature. Therefore our psychological knowledge should be based with the spiritual foundation.

Man, however obscure he may be now, has still a spirit in him. The spirit uses the mind, life and body for an individual and communal experience and manifests in the universe. This spirit is an infinite existence limiting itself apparently in the individual. This spirit is an infinite consciousness which defines itself in finite forms for the joy of various knowledge and power. This spirit is infinite delight of being which is trying to expand itself in various ways of joy. Therefore, the spirit in man is eternal Sachchidananda. And to reveal the infinite in the finite form of man, is the real goal of our life. This revelation of the Spirit is visible through the divine eye.

## Development of the Divine Eye

For the development of the divine eye it is necessary that our mind should be purified and a new consciousness should emerge in it.

The seat of mind or human consciousness is the brain. Unless the brain substance is changed there can be no change in the consciousness and in the movements of the external life; there can be no divine vision, the truth of things cannot be grasped, the hidden divine cannot be seen.

The brain consists of three parts:

1. Cerebrum
2. Cerebellum
3. Medula

**Cerebrum** is the seat of intellect and intelligence. Its topmost portion, the crown, is usually associated with the higher functions of mind, tending towards intuition, direct knowledge, luminous vision etc. The forehead is the seat of intellect proper, the rational mind, will andvision.

**Cerebellum** is usually associated with vital urges, impulsions, sentiments, passions, desires, etc.; the nervous centres, in the cerebellum control the lower functions of the mind. It is a control room for all dynamic actions and character and nature.

**Medula** is usually associated with the lower impulses, the demands and needs of the bodily functions.

Now the question is how to purify the mind or brain so that a new functioning may start and the old order of organisation may change and one may see the divine in every thing. There are two methods:

1. **Descent**—By the descent of Light and Power from above

into the brain substance. Through our aspiration the Light
will descend so as to penetrate into the brain and work out
the process of purification and develop new vision and new
organisation. This method has its limitations, hence the divine
eye is developed partially. The higher light descends but cannot penetrate far below into the brain. The cerebrum receives
the light comparatively easily: the cerebellum is just touched,
but the medula, the bottom portion of the brain is rarely contac-
ted. In other words, the intellect and intelligence is somewhat
illumined with a new light from above and even the higher
vital is also influenced, but the lower vital hardly gets its
touch. And the lowest region of physical movements remains
almost undisturbed.

2. **Ascent**—A force of fire is rocketed upwards and made
to strike at the lower portions of the brain. This secret fire,
the force of living flame is coiled and concentrated at the base
of the spine of the human system. This Kundalini, this energy
is forceful and fierce; its awakening can cause destruction to
the ignorant and ambitious, but for the aspirant and awakened
soul it works as the immortalising nectar.

The energy at the root of the spine is stored in the Muladhara
or the material centre. It is the concentrated energy in matter
something like a tree in the seed or atomic energy in the
stone. When this material energy is kindled, it moves upwards
piercing the different centres or chakras of the body and reaches
the head, and then goes beyond to join the supreme light and
force. As a result of the ascent there is descent of the light
and force from above into the lowest regions of the brain. So
this flaming force hidden in the material centre will do the
final work of purification of the brain by calling the Light from
above. By the descent of this supramental Light the consciousness of man will be changed, the divine eye will be fully

developed, God will be visible in everything and everywhere.

**How to Awaken this Kundalini?** When there is intense aspiration in the body then it is kindled, it is awakened by the pressure and fire of aspiration.


THE END